1976

ECOLOGICAL ANIMAL PARASITOLOGY

Ecological Animal Parasitology

C. R. KENNEDY B.Sc., Ph.D.

Department of Biological Sciences
University of Exeter

A HALSTED PRESS BOOK

JOHN WILEY & SONS

NEW YORK

© 1975 Blackwell Scientific Publications
Osney Mead, Oxford,
85 Marylebone High Street, London W1M 3DE.
9 Forrest Road, Edinburgh,
P.O. Box 9, North Balwyn, Victoria, Australia.

First published 1975

Published in the U.S.A. by
Halsted Press, a Division of
John Wiley & Sons, Inc.,
New York

Library of Congress Cataloging in Publication Data

Kennedy, Clive Russell, 1941—
    Ecological animal parasitology.

"A Halsted Press book."
Bibliography: p.
Includes index.

1. Parasitology. 2. Host-parasite relationships.
3. Zoology–Ecology. I. Title. [DNLM: 1. Parasite QX4 J37e].

QL757.K46   591.5'24   75–5760
ISBN 0–470–46910–2

Printed in Great Britain

Contents

Preface

There exist at present numerous texts on general parasitology but few devoted specifically to ecological parasitology and designed for an undergraduate readership. The aim of this book is to remedy this situation and to present and interpret animal parasitology in the light of some current ecological ideas and concepts. It is intended primarily for undergraduates, as a text to accompany a unit course on ecological parasitology or to supplement and complement courses on parasitology with other approaches. It is hoped, however, that it will also be of interest to students in other branches of zoology.

The approach adopted by the author is that of an ecologist, and because of that the more traditional approach to parasitology of describing the anatomy, physiology and life cycles of parasites in detail is avoided. These aspects are adequately treated in other books, and some basic knowledge of them is assumed. It is hoped that the selection of examples will compensate for any deficiencies in knowledge, and a brief summary of the classification and life cycles of the most important parasites considered in the text is provided in an appendix for the convenience of readers. This book concentrates instead upon the population biology of parasites. It aims to show how host and parasite interact at the population level, and discusses the factors that determine the size of parasite populations and the establishment, maintainance and control of host-parasite systems. It must be emphasised here that the author is not attempting an inter-disciplinary synthesis of parasitology and ecology. Whilst recognising both the value and magnitude of such a task, he is happy to leave it to someone more competent to execute it.

Little of the information contained in this book is new or previously unpublished since it is the approach that is considered important. As in any book, the author has had to be selective. The selection reflects in part his interests and in part the information available. This particular book makes no attempt to be comprehensive. It deals only with animal parasites, and bacteria and viruses are specifically excluded. Even amongst animal parasites, helminths are emphasised and insects and other arthropods receive little attention. This is only partly because they do not fall directly into the area of the author's own interests. The author believes that insect-host relationships are rather different from other parasite-host ones. Because of their greater mobility, their greater searching range and their different strategy, parasitic insects are more similar to predators than to other parasites, and so are excluded from this book. They are also treated in some detail in some excellent recent books. Instead, examples have been selected as far as possible on the basis of their inherent suitability, and if this has resulted in a bias towards some groups, then this reflects the current state of knowledge of animal parasitology. It is hoped that the reader will supplement the examples with others drawn from his own areas of interest and knowledge. If, as the author believes, the principles are applicable to the whole field of animal parasitology, then this should present little difficulty.

C.R.Kennedy

Acknowledgements

I am very grateful to Dr R.Avery and Dr J.C.Chubb for reading this book in manuscript and commenting critically upon it and making many useful suggestions as to content and presentation. I am also indebted to the many people with whom I have discussed my ideas and parts of the text: in particular I would single out for mention the late Dr H.D.Crofton, Prof. O.Halvorsen, Dr A.Rumpus and Miss E.Towner. Above all, I should like to thank my wife for her continual encouragement.

All the illustrations have been drawn or re-drawn from original sources by Mrs P.Broughton. I should like to thank her for her care and skill with this task, and for interpreting my instructions so well.

All the drawings which are not original are adapted from sources which are acknowledged in the accompanying legends. I am indebted to the following publishers for permission to reproduce illustrations: Cambridge University Press for Figs 5, 6, 7, 8, 10, 13, 15, 17, 18, 20, 23, 24, 29, 31, 32, 34, and 35 from *Parasitology*; McGraw-Hill Book Company for Fig. 1 from *Biological Control Systems Analysis* by J.H.Milsum; The Royal Society for Fig. 11 from *Proceedings of the Royal Society, Series B*; Academic Press Inc. for Fig. 12 from *Experimental Parasitology* and Fig. 30 from *Advances in Parasitology*; Blackwell Scientific Publications Ltd. for Figs 9, 22, and 28 from *Symposia of the British Society for Parasitology*; The Wildfowl Trust for Fig. 25 from *Wildfowl*; Appleton-Century-Crofts for Fig. 26 from *Immunity to Parasitic Animals*, edited by G.J.Jackson, R.Herman and J.Singer; Adam Hilger Ltd. for Fig. 27 from *Ecology and Physiology of Parasites* edited by A.M.Fallis; The Royal Society of Tropical Medicine and Hygiene for Fig. 33 from *Transactions of the Royal Society of Tropical Medicine and Hygiene*; Taylor and Francis Ltd. for Fig. 16 from the *Journal of Natural History*.

1 Introduction

THE NATURE OF PARASITISM

Ecological animal parasitology is concerned with the distribution and abundance of parasites. This includes their distribution and abundance in space, in time and in different hosts, and involves consideration of the factors regulating host-parasite interactions at both the individual and the population level. It is above all concerned with the quantitative as well as qualitative relationships between parasites and their hosts. It is necessary therefore to be clear not only what is meant by a parasitic relationship but also to try and express this in quantitative terms.

In view of the difficulties of trying to delimit a relationship that is not discrete but which merges into other interspecific relationships it is clearly difficult to define parasitism precisely. Instead it is possible and more useful to recognise the characteristics of the relationship, the most important of which is that it is a relationship between two species populations. The essential features of it have been expressed clearly by Crofton (1971a). These are that the parasite is physiologically dependent upon the host, that it has a higher reproductive potential than the host, that it is capable ultimately of killing heavily infected hosts, and that the infection process tends to produce an overdispersed distribution of parasites within the host population. Overdispersion is used here to describe the situation in which the distribution of the parasite population throughout that of its host is not random but in which the majority of parasites are found in relatively few host individuals. The mean number of parasites per host is less than its variance, and the frequency distribution of the parasites on or within their hosts can be described by a mathematical model suitable for aggregated distributions such as the Negative Binomial.

Although many objections can be raised to this as a definition of parasitism, especially the fact that many parasites never appear under natural conditions to reach a level at which they do kill their host, this approach to parasitism focuses attention upon a number of very important features of the parasitic relationship. These are that the host and parasite interact at both the individual and the population level, that this interaction can be quantified, and that for survival of the parasite population only a very few host individuals, those carrying the heavy infections, may be important.

PARASITE POPULATION GROWTH

The population of a parasite is considered to comprise all the individuals of that parasite species within a particular area, regardless of whether some of the

1

individuals are free-living or are located in or on a host at any one moment. The terms parasite burden and level of infection are used to refer to that part of the population which, at any particular time, is located in the host population.

Because of their complex life histories involving generally a low probability of locating and establishing within a host parasites have very high reproductive rates. If all the individuals survived the parasites would greatly outnumber the hosts, with potential danger to the latter. When the host and parasite populations are in equilibrium, the net reproductive rate of the parasites must be 1. To maintain this equilibrium when either the population density of the host changes or conditions favouring the survival of the parasite alter, the parasite must be able to adjust its reproductive rate or its mortality rate in relation to that of its host. Overinfection of hosts must always be a potential danger to parasites. No population overexploiting its resources is likely to survive, and the host provides all the essential resources of food and space for the parasite. If, furthermore, the parasite is capable of directly or indirectly increasing the mortality rate of the host population then for a stable host-parasite relationship to persist overinfection must be avoided and the population density of the parasite regulated in relation to that of the host. In the absence of such regulation the relationship can only be stable for short periods when a particular combination of the factors controlling the density of both host and parasite populations occurs fortuitously. At other times controls will operate on both populations independently of each other, and the relationship will necessarily be unstable. Stability is used here and throughout this book to refer to the ability of any population or system to come to an equilibrium, and to return to that equilibrium or to a new equilibrium level if perturbed.

The growth of a parasite population, like that of the population of any free-living animal, would, if unchecked, continue exponentially. It could thus be described by the general equation for exponential population growth (see Wilson and Bossert, 1971, for a discussion of the derivation of this equation):

$$\frac{dP}{dt} = rP$$

where P is the population size, dP/dt is the calculus notation for the rate of increase of P with time, and r is a constant called the intrinsic rate of increase of the population.

In a few situations, for example the build up of nematode infections in lambs in spring and early summer, the parasite population does increase exponentially. This happens, however, for only a short period and the increase is checked. This is true also of populations in general. The exponential phase of their increase persists for only a short time, and checks on the growth then begin to operate. These checks may be of two distinct types. They may operate equally effectively over the whole range of population densities, or they may operate with increasing severity as the population size increases. They need not be mutually exclusive, and checks of both types may operate on a population. Only the latter type, however, can result in a stable system, and it necessitates an addition to the equation above of some term which indicates the resistance to population growth as a function of population size. The equation thus becomes the logistic equation for population growth:

$$\frac{dP}{dt} = rP \left(\frac{K-P}{K}\right)$$

where K is the value of P when birth rate equals death rate and the population maintains a stable size. This indicates that the rate of growth slows down as the population size increases in a manner directly related to the population size until a state of equilibrium is reached. Checks of the former type, unrelated in severity to population density, will only produce an unstable equilibrium.

THE HOST AND PARASITE AS A SYSTEM

An alternative approach to the problems created by the growth of parasite populations is to view them in terms of general systems theory. This employs a basic universal model of a system (a 'black box') with an input and an output. These are designated by incoming and outgoing arrows to represent the relevant variables (Fig. 1A). The model is capable of further and more detailed elaboration as required, and any system can be broken down into smaller systems if necessary. Since systems theory is particularly concerned with time-varying or dynamic situations it is especially helpful in describing and analysing biological situations (Milsum, 1967). A further advantage of such models is that they can be constructed on a qualitative basis to describe information flow, control factors and the points at which they act or on a quantitative basis, where the terms are replaced by mathematical expressions. In the latter case computors may be used to simulate the real system and study the quantitative effects of the component variables upon output (Chapter 10). If, then, the parasite population is considered as a dynamic system, its growth can be represented in a systems model (Fig. 1B). In this case there is no true independent input variable, but only the initial parasite population, P_o. Where r is positive there is clearly a circulating effect causing growth to continue and producing the exponential rise in population. This circulating effect is known as a positive-feedback loop. This is considered positive because it causes the population to depart further and further from its original steady state of equilibrium. Positive feedback nearly always produces unstable systems, and as such is rarely encountered in biological control systems.

Instead, the more common control system is negative feedback. This is represented in its simplest form in Fig. 1B. The number of larvae entering a host is considered as the input, and the number of eggs produced by adults developing from those larvae as the output. The system itself, the host, and parasites within it, are broken into smaller boxes to show the stages in control more clearly. If the system is to remain in equilibrium, then the output must be related to the input. The input is thus not only the basic input but also the required input, and egg production must be controlled in such a way that it will continue to generate this input. This is best understood if it is assumed that there

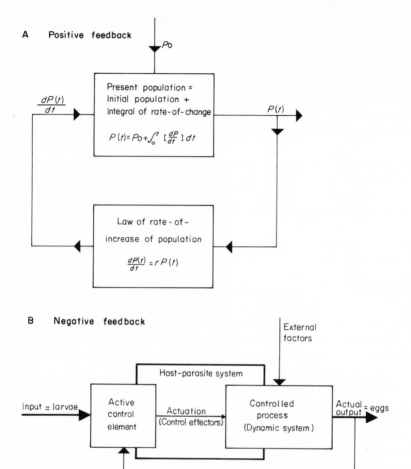

A   Positive feedback

P_0

$$\frac{dP(t)}{dt}$$

Present population =
Initial population +
Integral of rate-of-change

$$P(t) = P_0 + \int_0^t \left[\frac{dP}{dt}\right] dt$$

$P(t)$

Law of rate-of-
increase of population

$$\frac{dP(t)}{dt} = r P(t)$$

B   Negative feedback

External factors

Host-parasite system

Input = larvae

Active control element

Actuation
(Control effectors)

Controlled process
(Dynamic system)

Actual output = eggs

Feedback of output

Fig. 1 Block diagrams for population models showing information flow. (After Milsum, 1967.)

is no mortality in the egg stage. In this case the output must directly equal the input. This is brought about by monitoring the output in a feedback path for comparison with the input in a control element. If there is a difference, or error, between them, the control element acts upon the system, causing the actual output value to become closer to that of the desired output, in this example the input, and so reduce the error. Environmental changes or disturbances can be incorporated into the system at the point indicated. This feedback control is considered negative because it tends to restore the population to its original steady equilibrium state. Thus, negative feedback produces stable systems, and is widely encountered as a control mechanism throughout the whole range of biological systems. In the equation for population growth $(K-P/K)$ is an indication of negative feedback, since it acts to produce a steady population size.

4

CONTROLS AND STABILITY OF HOST-PARASITE SYSTEMS

If, therefore, the density of a parasite population is to be regulated in relation to that of its host to prevent overcrowding and produce a stable system then negative feedback control must be employed. This need not be the only control, nor need it operate all the time. In the course of their life cycle parasites will be exposed to many potential mortality factors, including climate and inability to locate a host when they possess limited food reserves and so have a short life span, and these may depress and maintain the population at a level where overcrowding of hosts is impossible and feedback controls never actually operate. Such a situation will nevertheless be unstable, and if the factors change and favour the parasite, then overcrowding may again present a danger. In these circumstances negative feedback controls may come into operation. If they are to control the parasite in relation to its host, then they must operate at that stage of the life cycle of the parasite when the parasite and host come into contact. Regulation of the parasite population size in any habitat must thus be achieved through regulation of numerous and separate individual host-parasite relationships and infection levels.

Several features of this relationship can serve as feedback controls. These could involve the behaviour of the parasite population itself, by way of overcrowding leading to reduced growth rate and egg production. They could also involve the host response. If the parasite burden in a host rises above a threshold value (Dineen, 1963) then the host may respond to the parasite immunologically, causing a variety of effects upon the parasites including expulsion of all or part of them from the host, reduced egg production and retardation of larval development. Low parasite burdens would, however, be tolerated and would evoke no such response. All these controls could operate simultaneously or sequentially as the parasite burden rises. In either event, there is no reason to suppose that there exists only a single feedback control for any host-parasite relationship.

Very similar conclusions were reached by Bradley (1974) in an attempt to understand the basis for the stability of many parasite populations. He considered that there were three basic ways of controlling parasite populations:

(1). The first of these was by transmission of the parasite. Small changes in transmission rate could lead to large changes in population size. Such changes are, however, greatly affected by independent factors such as climate, and unless transmission rate is related in some way to population density and so can operate in a feedback manner, this control by environmental factors would be imperfect and lead to erratic fluctuations in parasite population size since the system would be unstable.

(2). Where transmission was more effective, parasite numbers could increase by asexual reproduction or addition until they severly affected or killed the hosts. The death of hosts at high population densities would reduce transmission rates, and damage to the host population would be minimised by over-dispersion of the parasites so that only a proportion of the host population would be killed. This heterogeneity would result in a degree of regulation of parasite numbers, since host, and therefore parasite, mortality would be dependent upon parasite density, and would tend to stabilise the system.

(3). Stability could also be achieved by host responses as discussed above, since these are dependent in extent upon the parasite burden. Thus when the transmission levels necessary for persistence of the parasite population are exceeded, mechanisms for stabilising the population and the host-parasite system often come into operation.

Because these controls involve the host as well as the parasite, and indeed regulation of the parasite population may be achieved entirely by the host, it is evident that the host and parasite must be considered as a single system for many purposes. This ability of the system to regulate itself would protect both host and parasite and contribute to a stable, though dynamic, relationship. The threshold tolerated and the vigour of the response will vary, both between host individuals of one species and between hosts of different species, depending on the virulence of the parasite and the condition and suitability of the host. In the course of the evolution of a host-parasite system, however, selection for negative feedback controls would be expected since, together with selection for immunological disparity between the parasite and host, it would result in a stable relationship.

This concept of stability is more applicable at the population than at the individual level, and its achievement does not imply that all individual host-parasite relationships are also stable. Within any population hosts may show genetically based variation in susceptibility to parasitic infection, and parasites in infectivity. This may be accentuated by the over-dispersed distribution of the parasites within the host population, such that in only some individuals is the threshold beyond which a response is provoked exceeded. The response tends in fact to depend upon quantitative rather than mere qualitative information. The effects of the parasites upon some host individuals may thus be severe and lead to their death, and the individual relationships be very unstable. Nevertheless, the populations of both the hosts and the parasites will persist and may be quite stable.

2 Dispersal and location of hosts

GENERAL CONSIDERATIONS

Dispersal away from the parent individual or from the centre of the population in order to ensure survival of the species by colonising new areas and by preventing overcrowding with its resultant mortality is necessary for all animals, and particularly for parasites because of the continual danger of their overinfecting their hosts. All parasites or their reproductive products must therefore be capable of escaping from their hosts and locating new ones. The new hosts may be members of the same generation as the old ones, but there may also be a specific need for the parasite to transfer from one host generation to the next. In either case, some stage of a parasite's life cycle is very often spent outside of any hosts. This stage is the one that frequently accomplishes dispersal, but because the probability of finding a new host is generally very low, mortality amongst dispersal stages may be very high. To compensate for this, parasite fecundity may be very high also and asexual reproduction is of frequent occurrence.

Free-living stages create additional problems, since the parasite has to adapt to two dissimilar sets of conditions, those inside and those outside the host. In addition, therefore, to dispersing in space parasites may also have to be capable of dispersing in time, and of surviving periods of unfavourable climatic conditions until such time as they improve or the parasites locate a new host. This may be achieved by the incorporation of an inactive, protected resting stage into the life cycle or by the incorporation of another host, or by both. They both remove the parasite to some extent from the dangers of climatic fluctuations and extend its range in time, but intermediate hosts also assist its dispersal by extending its range in space as a result of the hosts' activities, and, by virtue of the ecological links existing between intermediate and definitive hosts, direct it towards the latter. The behaviour of the parasites within the intermediate host or of the host itself may also be such as to increase the probability of locating the definitive host. The details of each life cycle depend upon the hosts employed, and variations are typically related to problems of transfer, timing and synchronisation of host and parasite cycles in order to ensure survival to the next generation.

FECUNDITY OF PARASITES

EGG PRODUCTION

The high fecundity of parasites is generally held to be one of their most characteristic features, and to be associated with the heavy mortality in the course of dispersal. In practice however precise estimates are very difficult to obtain, and frequently relate only to one stage in the life history. Figures for egg output give some idea of the potential. A single female of the large roundworm *Ascaris lumbricoides* can produce 200,000 eggs per day for a year, of *Haemonchus contortus* 10,000 eggs per day and of *Litomosoides carinii* 15,000 microfilariae per day. *Fasciola hepatica*, the liver fluke, may produce 20,000 eggs per day and over 1,000,000 eggs in the course of its life, and a single adult *Taenia saginata,* the beef tapeworm, 100,000 eggs per day or 50–150 million in a year. Where the parasite is capable of asexual reproduction at some stage in its life history fecundity is further increased. It is virtually impossible to make accurate estimates for protozoans, many of which have at least one stage of asexual reproduction, but 1 oocyst of *Eimeria tenella* can theoretically produce 2.5 million second generation merozooites. Amongst digeneans, a single mother sporocyst of a plagiorchid may produce 3–4000 daughter sporocysts, and of a strigeid 4000 rediae. Large snails parasitised by *Echinostoma revolutum* may contain up to 1724 rediae per snail. Numbers may be further increased by cercarial production. A single miracidium of *F. hepatica* may produce over 600 cercariae. A single *Littorina littorea* infected by *Cryptocotyle lingua* emitted up to 3300 cercariae per day, and 1,300,000 in its first year. It continued production, although at a reduced rate, for five years.

There can be no doubt therefore that many parasites do have an enormous fecundity. As Cole (1954) has pointed out, fecundity is also related to the age at which the parasite commences to breed. The biotic potential of a species is increased as the length of the pre-reproductive part of the life span is decreased, and this may be just as important to a high fecundity as the number of progeny produced per day. Repeated reproduction on the part of the parasite may also be an advantage, in that it does not overtax the parasite's resources and disperses the eggs more widely in time as well as space. Where reproduction is confined to a very short period and the reproductive phase of the life cycle is very short it is often found that the life histories of both host and parasite have to be synchronised very closely.

ASEXUAL REPRODUCTION

Fecundity is often enhanced by the occurrence of asexual reproduction in the course of a life cycle. This can take place by a variety of methods, from simple division amongst some protozoans and budding in cestodes to the unique processes amongst digeneans that result in cercarial production. Amongst trypanosomes it is the only method of reproduction. It may occur in the definitive host or in the intermediate host or vector, or in both, or even in a resting stage outside of the host. In some species, notably of *Plasmodium*, the malaria parasite, more than one cycle of asexual reproduction may take place within a single host. The occurrence of asexual reproduction does not correlate with habitat, nor the method adopted with the status of the host in the life cycle or the type of life cycle itself. In some cases, especially that of cercarial production, it may be associated with the dispersal of the parasite and the change of hosts, but equally often dispersal is accomplished by the sexual products.

Asexual reproduction must therefore be regarded as a further method of increasing parasite fecundity and thus ensuring the continued survival of the parasite population under conditions where there is a low probability of any individual establishing and reproducing (Cole, 1954). Thus, amongst digeneans, the heavy mortality in the miracidial stage and the low probability of infecting a snail is counteracted to some extent by the ability of the few miracidia that do infect snails to reproduce asexually. This has inevitable consequences with regard to both life tables (p. 11) and parasite dispersion (p. 68), since the presence of one parasite individual within a single host must lead inevitably to the presence of others. It may also be considered adaptive in that it allows for greatly increased reproduction during periods when conditions for the parasite are favourable and resources adequate. Because it perpetuates existing genotypes it also contributes towards the population isolation and strain formation found amongst so many parasites (Chapter 3).

GENERATION TIME

Estimates of egg and larval production must be considered not only in terms of the length of the reproductive period but also in terms of the generation time. A single female of *Haemonchus contortus* can produce 10,000 eggs per day, of which 5000 are potential females. The generation time in this species, i.e. the time for an egg to develop into a mature female, is one month (see Appendix for life cycle). Assuming no mortality, after three months this one female would have given rise to 10^{11} females. Equivalent reproductive rates may, however, be attained with the production of far fewer eggs providing the generation time is also reduced (Crofton, 1966). From Table 1 it can be seen that a female producing only 20 eggs in its life span may have the same reproductive potential as *H. contortus* providing its generation time is as short as one week. A low rate of

Table 1 Reproductive rates equivalent to that of *H. contortus*. (From Crofton, 1966.)

Generation time (days)	No. of eggs produced per female
3	5
5	9
7	20
14	200
21	2,000

egg production is therefore usually associated with a short generation time, whereas the production of large numbers of eggs is usually accompanied by a longer generation time. This latter pattern is commonly encountered amongst parasites, but so are other patterns, and estimates of egg production not accompanied by information on generation times mean very little.

A further difficulty encountered in estimating parasite fecundity is that neither the rate of egg production nor the generation time are constant. Egg production may decline naturally as the parasite becomes senescent, but it is also influenced strongly by the host's response to the parasite. Indeed, one of the characteristic features of host immune responses to parasites is a reduction in their rate of reproduction (Table 2), this functioning as a negative feedback control upon the size of the parasite population. The generation time is also variable since it depends upon climatic conditions, especially temperature (Table 3), and also upon host responses. Another characteristic feature of host

Table 2 The reproductive index (RI) for 4 species of *Eimeria* based on oocyst output following two successive infections. (From Horton-Smith and Long, 1963.)

Species	Details	After 1st infection	After 2nd infection	Ratio of indices
E. acervulina	Dose	500,000	500,000	
	RI	1,026	12	86:1
E. tenella	Dose	500	5,000	
	RI	64,000	4,600	14:1
E. necatrix	Dose	500	5,000	
	RI	12,000	1,360	9:1
E. maxima	Dose	500	5,000	
	RI	30,000	5.2	5700:1

Table 3 The effects of constant temperature on the development rate of eggs and larvae of five species of cattle nematodes. (From Ciordia and Bizzell, 1963.)

		Temperature °C							
		5	6	8	10	15	20	25	35
Median time	1st stage	28	32	21	17	10	5–7	5–7	2
(days) to	3rd stage	—	41	32	26–28	19	9	7–9	3
% of eggs infective		0	1.3	3.5	8.3	13.4	21.5	30	5.3

responses to nematodes is a retardation of their larval development at a particular stage. The larva survives but does not develop further until the response is reduced. By thus increasing the generation time, parasite fecundity is reduced and so the population size is controlled by the host. Each parasite species has in fact a basic characteristic fecundity, age at reproduction and generation time which, though variable, are adaptive and lead to a determined set of consequences (Cole, 1954).

LIFE TABLES

Although parasites are undoubtedly very fertile, it is difficult to make exact and meaningful determinations of their reproductive potential. Their great fecundity is a measure of the difficulties that they face and the enormous mortality that occurs in the completing of a life cycle when the probability of locating a host is very low. In order to appreciate fully both the high fecundity and mortality it would be necessary to examine the life tables of the parasites, but the information necessary for compiling these is seldom available. Very heavy mortality in the free living stages would be predicted, but with a very high survival rate when the parasite had invaded a host. This would be especially true where the parasite is capable of asexual reproduction, since even if only a single individual survives to infect a host it may nevertheless give rise to numerous progeny.

An attempt has been made by Hairston (1965) to construct life tables for schistosomes (Table 4) based on field data. Assuming that the host and parasite

Table 4 Life tables of human schistosome species. (From Hairston, 1965.)

	S. haematobium	*S. mansoni*	*S. japonicum*
Daily output of cercariae	900	3500	55
Net reproductive rate in snails	3163	11,252	63.3
Probability of successful infection by cercariae	9.22×10^{-5}	6.9×10^{-7}	4.3×10^{-6}(man) 1.0×10^{-5}(rats) 1.7×10^{-6}(dogs) 9.8×10^{-6}(pigs)
Net reproductive rate in man	26,743	11,493	90,471
Probability of successful infection by miracidia	5.04×10^{-4}	2.59×10^{-2}	2.31×10^{-2}

populations are in a state of equilibrium and the parasite population is constant from year to year, the net reproductive rate of the parasite must equal 1. Therefore

$$\text{net reproductive rate in snails} \times \text{probability of successfully infecting a mammal} \times \text{net reproductive rate in mammals} \times \text{probability of successful infection of a snail} = 1$$

All these rates and probabilities were estimated for the three species of schistosome infecting man. It is clear that as predicted probabilities of infection are very low, fecundity very high, and mortality at all stages in the life cycle very high. The low probability of a miracidium infecting a snail is compensated for by the high rate of asexual reproduction and large numbers of cercariae produced. Thus, although the complex life cycle achieves the successful dispersal of the parasites, it requires a very high reproductive potential.

DISPERSAL OF PARASITES

Parasite dispersal can be accomplished in several different ways and by employing different stages in the life cycle. Dispersal in time is frequently accomplished by the presence of a resting stage in the life cycle. Development of such a stage is halted and is not resumed until the parasite receives a specific stimulus that can often only be provided by its next host (p. 17). When the resting stages are free in the surrounding medium they are very resistant to changing and unfavourable climatic conditions, and are usually enclosed within a protective covering, which may be an egg capsule, an oocyst wall or the moulted skin of a previous larval stage. Free living resting stages are often immobile, and so only disperse the parasite in time and not space (Table 5). If the resting stage is passed within another host, then the movements of that host will also assist dispersal in space.

Table 5 Survival times of some parasite stages. (From various sources.)

Species	Stage	Condition	and	Site	Survival
Fasciola hepatica	miracidia	free living	in	water	c. 24h
Schistosoma douthitti	cercaria	free living	in	water	c. 11h
Triaenophorus nodulosus	coracidium	free living	in	water	c. 24h
Diphyllobothrium latum	eggs	free	in	water	months
Eimeria sp.	oocysts	free	on	pasture	c.6 months
Haemonchus contortus	larvae	encysted	on	pasture	c.6 months
Moniliformis hirudinaceus	ancanthors	free	in	soil	up to 3½ years
Trupansosoma sp.	in vector				as long as vector weeks → months
Diplostomum spathaceum	metacercaria			eye of fish	up to 5 years
Trianophorus nodulosus	pleroceroid			body cavity of fish	3 years

Dispersal in space is also accomplished by motile, free living larval stages such as ciliated spores, cercariae or nauplii. Such larvae seldom feed and so are short lived and subject to very heavy mortality (Table 5). Although they may be provided with cilia or other structures for locomotion they are seldom able to cover large distances by their own efforts. They rely far more on transport by other sources such as water currents. They may then cover quite considerable distances even within their short life span (Table 6), although the parasite burden acquired by hosts is inversely proportional to the distance the larvae are

Table 6 Worm burden of *Schistosoma mansoni* in mice exposed at various distances downstream of an experimental source of infection. (From Radke *et al.*, 1961.)

No. of cercariae per gallon	Feet downstream: 100	Mean number of worms per mouse				
		500	1000	1500	2000	2500
25	16	3	3	1	0.2	—
62	25	9	14	4	4.0	0.2
114	34	13	11	9	4.0	0.4

carried away from the source of infection and to the strength of the water current. Such stages also serve the important function of locating the new hosts (p. 18).

Dispersal of parasites in both time and space is also accomplished by the movements of the infected hosts themselves. Parasites can survive in some intermediate hosts for the whole life span of the latter. They may thus be distributed throughout an area by the movements of the host or vector alone. The movement of infected shrimps was considered by Hynes and Nicholas (1963) to be far more important to the dispersal of *Polymorphus minutus* than the passive drift of acanthors (Table 7). When adult, the movements of the definitive host within its habitat is effective in dispersing the eggs or cysts throughout the area, especially if they are not all produced upon a single occasion (p. 8).

Table 7 Infection of *Gammarus pulex* with *Polymorphus minutus* above and below a duck pen on a small stream. (From Hynes and Nicholas, 1963.)

	Distance in metres from duck pen						
Above pen	300	50					
Below pen			10	250	800	2000	5000
% infected	3.0	15.1	70.9	62.9	85.3	56.4	15.6
Mean parasite burden	1.1	1.8	3.3	2.3	2.0	1.3	1.1

LOCATION OF HOSTS AND INFECTION

BY VECTORS

In cycles involving a vector, location of the host is accomplished by the vector and depends upon its behaviour and biting habits, and the detailed ecological relationships between the two hosts are utilised to effect infection. Amongst trypanosomes a range of transfer methods is employed. *Trypanosoma cruzi* employs biting bugs of the family Reduviidae as vectors, and its infective stages occur in the rectum of the bug. When it bites the vertebrate, trypanosomes are passed out with the faeces and infection is accomplished by the host rubbing the wound contaminated with the faeces. This method of infection is hence known as contaminative. The rat trypanosome, *T. lewisi*, uses a flea as its vector

(Appendix). Infection is again contaminative, by ingestion of flea faeces, but may also occur by crushing and ingestion of the flea in the course of grooming.

Trypanosoma gambiense, the cause of sleeping sickness in man, employs flies of the genus *Glossina,* the tsetse fly, as vectors, and its infective stages occur in the salivary glands of the fly. When the tsetse bites a vertebrate, the trypanosomes are injected into the blood stream via the proboscis (Appendix and Fig. 2). This

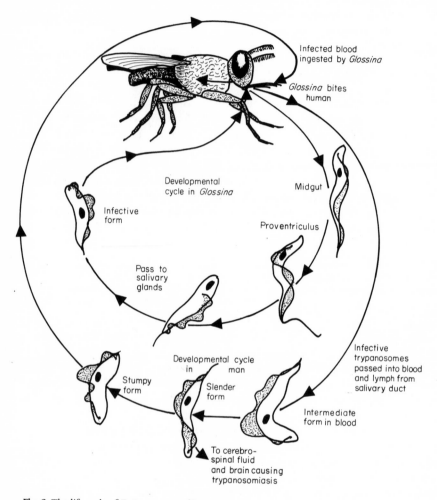

Fig. 2 The life cycle of *Trypanosoma gambiense.*

method of transmission is hence known as inoculative. In all these cases the trypanosomes survive for at least a matter of weeks in the vector and undergo development there. In some cases however transmission can be purely mechanical. In South America *T. vivax* employs flies of the genus *Tabanus* as vectors, but it undergoes no development in the fly and is infective only so long as the ingested blood is moist. Transmission thus depends on the fly being interrupted in the course of feeding on one host, flying off and settling rapidly on another.

The vectors of filarial nematodes are also particularly well suited to the successful transfer of the parasite by virtue of the close ecological relationships between the vector and definitive host. In Africa *Simulium damnosum,* the vector of *Onchocerca volvulus,* prefers to bite in the region of the hips and thighs. The microfilariae are injected into this region, the adults form nodules in the same region and the microfilariae produced in them congregate more densley in this region, thus increasing the chance of being picked up by the same vector but by no other. In America, where flies bite in the head region, the microfilariae also congregate in the head region. In chimpanzees *O. gutterosa* is injected into the umbilical region, but the adults develop in the neck. The microfilariae therefore migrate back to the umbilicus where 90% of the flies bite.

BY INTERMEDIATE HOSTS AND RESTING STAGES

Where intermediate hosts are employed in the life cycle, location of the next host is not dependent upon any activity on the part of the parasite. The identity of the host it is in, its behaviour within it, and any effect it may have on it to render it more attractive to the next host will improve the probability of infection. It is, however, dependent upon the feeding habits of the next host, over which it has no control, for entry into it. Once in the correct intermediate host, however, the structure and trophic links of the food web in the habitat imposes upon the parasite a limited set of possibilities and consequences. It is in effect canalised, and so can only proceed along certain channels, so that the probability of its encountering its correct definitive host is greatly improved. It does not select or locate its next host as such, but it does have to recognise it as a potential host. If the parasite finds itself within a host which is unsuitable, it may pass straight out of it again or survive for a while before dying as a result of unfavourable conditons.

There is, however, another possibility, that the parasite will incorporate the host as a paratenic host. These arise by animals other than the normal hosts ingesting larvae or infected intermediate hosts, an inevitable consequence of animals having wide diets. In contrast to true definitive hosts or intermediate hosts which are obligatory in the life cycle, these are facultative, and the parasites never develop within them but merely survive whilst still remaining infective to the next host. They can never replace an intermediate host, but may interpose at any stage in the life cycle (Fig. 3). Their importance depends upon the importance of the food links between the hosts, and they may or may not facilitate transfer to the final host. Pike can serve as paratenic hosts in the life cycle of *Diphyllobothrium latum,* the broad tapeworm of man, and because the final host, man, actively selects large piscivorous fish, they do in this case facilitate transfer. The final hosts of *D. dendriticum* are, by contrast, birds, which select smaller fish rather than large pisciverous ones, and hence paratenic hosts are less important to the species (Halvorsen and Wissler, 1973). They are still advantageous in that mortality of parasites is reduced, dispersal in space is assisted, and dispersal in time is facilitated by their acting as an accumulator of parasites.

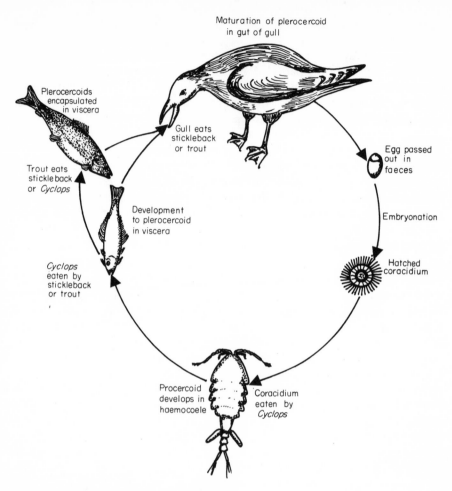

Fig. 3 The life cycle of *Diphyllobothrium dendriticum*.

Development of the larva within an intermediate host is, as noted previously, often suspended and is dependent upon a stimulus for resumption. Recognition of a suitable host, in so far as it occurs at all, is accomplished by receipt of this stimulus. Such a mechanism ensures that the parasite does not develop prematurely in the host in which it is contained, or in an unsuitable host, but only under conditions in which it has a reasonable chance of further survival.

The precise nature of the stimulus varies between different parasite species, but the general conditions for excystation, hatching from eggs and ex-sheathment of larvae are remarkably similar. The conditions provided by the host activate the parasite, which then emerges as a result of its own activities. Emergence of sporozoites from *Eimeria* oocysts only takes place following mechanical abrasions during passage through the gizzard of a bird and in the presence of CO_2, trypsin and bile (Hammond, 1971). Hatching of *Ascaris lumbricoides* eggs requires a temperature of 37°C, the presence of the appropriate concentration of dissolved gaseous CO_2, the correct redox potential and a pH of around 7.3 (Rogers, 1962). Under these conditions the enclosed larva secretes a hatching fluid which contains lipase, chitinase and a protease and which destroys the egg shell from the inside, thus liberating the larvae. The hatching of cyclophyllidean eggs such as those of *Hymenolepis diminuta,* the rat tapeworm, requires mechanical damage, presumably brought about by the jaws of the beetle intermediate host, the presence of CO_2, undissociated $NaHCO_3$, and enzymes such as trypsin, (Voge and Berntzen, 1961). Activation of taeniid tapeworm embryos requires in addition the presence of bile, since their larval stage is spent in a vertebrate host.

Emergence and activation of hymenolepid cystacanths in a vertebrate host also requires bile salts, in addition to the presence of proteolytic enzymes and reducing conditions (Rothman, 1959). Ex-sheathment of nematode larvae requires very similar conditions (Rogers and Sommerville, 1963). The presence of undissociated H_2CO_3, dissolved CO_2, and reducing agents at a temperature of around 37°C and a pH of 7–8 causes the larva to produce an ex-sheathing fluid which attacks a weak area of the enclosing sheath. Excystment of *Fasciola hepatica* metacercarial cysts also requires the correct temperature, the presence of CO_2, reducing conditions and bile (Dixon, 1966). In a few cases the stimulus may be very simple. A rise in temperature to just below 40°C is sufficient to induce plerocercoid larvae of the tapeworm *Schistocephalus solidus* to resume development (Smyth, 1952).

In all these cases the necessary conditions are only likely to be encountered within another animal, and thus hatching or emergence is deferred until the parasite enters another host. The necessary stimuli may however be provided by a number of animal species with which the parasite makes contact but which may not prove to be suitable hosts. In only a few cases are the stimuli so specific that they are likely to be provided by only one or two species of host. Larvae of *Haemonchus contortus* require unusually high concentrations of CO_2 and H_2CO_3 for ex-sheathment, and these are only likely to be found in the rumen of herbivorous ungulates (Rogers and Sommerville, 1963). Cysts of the cestode *Echinococcus* are damaged by the presence of deoxycholic acid in high concentrations. Such conditions are found in the bile of hares, rabbits and sheep which are in any case unsuitable hosts, but not in the bile of dogs, cats and foxes, their normal hosts (Smyth, 1962). In most cases therefore this mechanism does not enable a parasite to recognise its host, but only ensures that the infective stage resumes development under conditions that are more likely to be supplied by that host.

BY FREE LIVING LARVAL STAGES

Where resting stages are free living but hatch to produce active infective larvae, the stimulus to hatching may again be such as to ensure that the larvae only emerge under suitable conditions where the probability of locating the next host is increased. Eggs of *F. hepatica* only hatch under the influence of bright sunlight. This stimulates the fully formed miracidia to produce a hatching fluid which attacks the capsule and together with osmotic pressure changes in the egg causes the larvae to emerge (Rowan, 1956; Wilson, 1967). This ensures that only fully formed miracidia hatch, and that they do so under conditions in which the larvae can exhibit the phototactic responses essential to the location of the snail host. The eggs of *Nematodirus spathiger,* a sheep nematode, are passed out of sheep in summer, but are unable to hatch until they have experienced long periods at cold temperatures (Crofton, 1963). This prevents hatching until spring, when susceptible lambs are available for infection. Hatching of the eggs of the monogenean *Entobdella soleae* (Appendix) is enhanced by the presence of mucus from the skin of its definitive host, the sole (Kearn, 1974), although mucus from other fish may have a similar effect. Where the resting stage is free living but does not produce active larvae, its ingestion by the next host is purely fortuitous.

When transfer between hosts is accomplished by active free living larval stages, location of the next host is to a large extent dependent upon the activities of the parasites themselves. The larvae may move around at random depending upon chance for encounters with potential hosts, but more frequently they exhibit characteristic behaviour patterns which increase the probability of contact between host and parasite and favour transmission. These may take the form of a general attraction to the habitat of the host, or of directed movements to bring it within the range of the host, or of specific taxes (Wright, 1971).

The responses of digenean miracidia and cercariae to environmental stimuli are generally similar to those of their hosts, and serve to bring both host and parasite together in the same region. Their behaviour has been reviewed by Cable (1972). Wright (1959, 1964, 1971) has shown that encounters between miracidia and hosts are seldom due to chance, but that there is a sequential pattern of host selection. The first stage is a response to physical stimuli that takes the parasite into the region of its host. Miracidia generally show positive phototaxis and negative geotaxis, which takes them towards the water surface where snails are more abundant. *Schistosoma japonicum* shows positive phototaxis to any light intensity at 15°C. Below this temperature the response is negatively phototactic, which dominates the negative geotaxis, and the larvae sink. This change in behaviour is paralleled by that of its molluscan host. The responses of *S. mansoni* are such as to bring it near the margins of a locality, where the hosts also congregate.

The second phase of the sequence consists of random movements which bring the larvae into the range of the hosts. This typically takes the form of long, sweeping lines with occasional turns (Wright, 1971). It also assists dispersal of the larvae.

The third stage in the sequence involves chemotaxis or other directed responses to stimuli produced by the snails. The type of response is very variable, ranging from increased speed of locomotion through increased rate of turning to specific taxes. Wright (1959) suggested that miracidia followed gradients, though not along a straight line, and Ulmer (1971) confirmed that miracidia of the digenean *Megalodiscus temperatus* reached the host more directly and in a shorter time if the snails were isolated to allow the stimulating agent to diffuse. Miracidia of *S. mansoni* swim with a devious, twisting course in the presence of *Biomphalaria glabrata*, a pattern characteristic of a response to an olfactory stimulus. They are attracted to the whole snail, and to extracts of the foot, glands, faeces and water in which the snails have been kept (Wright, 1964, 1966a). They are less attracted to snail mucus or blood, despite the fact that Wright (1959) showed the existence of differences between the mucus of different species of snails. The stimulus is not very specific, as *S. mansoni* miracidia could respond to water conditioned by the presence of species of *Lymnea* as well as by species of *Biomphalaria*. MacInnis (1965) has shown that the attractants are some of the short-chain fatty acids and some of the amino acids of the host (Table 8).

Table 8 The attractiveness of amino acids to miracidia of *Schistosoma mansoni*. (From MacInnis, 1965.)

Acid	Butyric	Sialic	Glutamic	Valeric	Butyric + Sialic	Butyric + Glutamic	Control: no acid
% 'attracted'	69	65	65	61	69	50	5

It has also been shown that miracidia of *F. hepatica* are attracted to snail mucus, and that short-chain fatty acids influence their turning behaviour (Wilson, 1968; Wilson and Denison, 1970). Oncomiracidia of the monogenean *Entobdella soleae* are also able to respond to specific substances secreted by the skin of their host, and attach to sole skin in preference to that of related species and of other flatfish (Kearn, 1967).

The cercariae by contrast do not appear to be attracted specifically to their hosts. Instead they exhibit behaviour that brings them into the same region as the host, and most show positive phototaxis and negative geotaxis that brings them to the water surface. Some species may show more specific responses (Wright, 1971). Many amphistomes are attracted to green surfaces and so to marginal vegetation, whilst strigeids exhibit a shadow response whereby their activity increases and they swim upwards in response to a shadow. Such behaviour will increase the probability of their making contact with a fish. Some xiphidocercariae by contrast show negative phototaxis, a pattern that brings them into the same region as the benthic arthropods, their next host. Having encountered their host, schistosomes at least are able to recognise skin and require the presence of host lipids in order to stimulate penetration (Table 9).

The movements of nematode larvae are not easy to interpret. Strongyles move out of the faeces in a random manner, and most species then undergo vertical migrations. It appears that taxes may also be involved in some cases, especially phototaxes and geotaxes, but no evidence has yet been found of specific taxes towards animal hosts (Croll, 1972). In the course of their migration they select particular sites where they then remain. Those species that require to be eaten for transfer move onto blades of grass, whilst those that infect by penetration remain at the base of the vegetation where they are unlikely to be eaten. The activity of these species may increase when the temperature is raised,

Table 9 Evaluation of skin surface lipid as a cercarial penetration stimulus for *Schistosoma mansoni*. (From Stirewelt, 1971.)

Skin	Schistosomule collection average %	Cercarial penetration response
Untreated skin membrane	59	100
Membrane with skin lipid removed	4	2
Treated membrane + skin lipid	18	100
Brudruche membrane	0	0
Brudruche membrane + skin lipid	0	100

which would assist them to contact a warm-blooded grazing animal (Croll, 1972).

In general, apart from miracidia, specific taxes appear to be uncommon. Nevertheless, all larval stages behave in a manner that favours transmission. Since these active larvae have limited life spans the wastage must be enormous, and accounts for the high fecundity and extensive powers of asexual reproduction. The employment of an intermediate host or vector appears, by virtue of its directional component, to provide a more reliable method of host location, and it is perhaps for this reason that intermediate hosts are such a common feature of parasite life cycles. Intermediate hosts are also of benefit if temporary extinction of the parasites in the definitive host occurs for some reason, such as the disappearance of the host or unfavourable conditions for transmission, since they permit continuation of one stage of the parasite's life history and so persistence of the parasite population.

LIFE CYCLE FEATURES IMPROVING THE PROBABILITY OF INFECTION

BEHAVIOUR OF INFECTED HOSTS

Even though the mere inclusion of an intermediate host in the life cycle may increase the probability of the parasite locating the definitive host, the activities of the infected hosts themselves may increase the likelihood of their being acquired by the definitive host. Parasites have modified host behaviour in relation to several different predation strategies (Holmes and Bethel, 1972), and thus increased the vulnerability of infected hosts to predation. Cutaneous leishmaniasis, produced by *Leishmania tropica,* is characterised by the presence of sores and ulcers on the skin. Their presence attracts the vectors, anthropophilic sand flies, to those precise regions of the skin where the chances of picking up the parasites are greatest. A rather similar situation arises in infections by the nematode *Dracunculus medinensis,* the guinea worm. The mature females migrate to the surface layers of the skin, especially to areas that are likely to come into contact with water. A secretion of the parasite causes at first a blister and later a small ulcer. On contact with water larvae are released through the ulcer by projection of the uterus of the nematode. On removal from water the exposed part of the uterus dries and so inhibits release of further larvae. The intermediate host is a cyclopoid copepod, and this mechanism ensures that larvae are only released into the water where they may encounter the host.

Many species of Digenea have profound effects upon their host's behaviour. *Leucochloridium paradoxum* sporocysts, containing encysted cercariae, migrate to the tentacles of the snail host. They are brightly coloured, with red or green bands, and render the snail very conspicuous. In daylight they pulsate, whereas at night they withdraw into the snail body. In addition, infected snails, instead of being sheltered by the vegetation, crawl to the tips of leaves thus further increasing their conspicuousness and the probability of their being noticed by a bird. Metacercariae of *Dicrocoelium dentriticum*, the lancet fluke, encyst in ants. Of all those infecting the host, only one or two, usually the first to arrive, move to the host's brain and encyst in the suboesophageal ganglia. The behaviour of the infected ants is then modified, in that they move to the tip of the grass stems. At cold temperatures infected ants grasp the grass with their mandibles, and become torpid so that they are unable to drop off. The behaviour thus serves to keep infected animals exposed to the host at grazing times.

Parasites clearly modify host behaviour in order to be ingested by particular hosts, and this may involve not only increasing their conspicuousness so that the predator will select it in preference to uninfected animals, but also reducing the stamina or responses of the host. Strigeid metacercariae live in the eyes of fish, where they may cause complete or partial blindness. In either event, the normal pattern of fish behaviour is altered, and its normal responses slowed or inhibited. The presence of the cestode *Ligula* in fish not only renders them more conspicuous but also, by distorting their body, slows their speed. They also move into shallow water where they are even more obvious. Holmes and Bethel (1972) have shown that shrimps infected with *Polymorphus paradoxus* actively prefer the lighter areas and show positive photoaxis. They cling to floating vegetation, and grip onto the reed fragments at the water surface. Their hosts, mallard ducks, are attracted to such floating vegetation and so eat infected gammarids in preference to uninfected ones (Table 10), which normally live near

Table 10 Vulnerability of gammarids infected with *Polymorphus paradoxus* to predation by mallard ducks. (From Holmes and Bethel, 1972.)

		Gammarids eaten		
Test no.	Duck no.	Uninfected	Infected	
1	2	*6/25	16/25	
2	2	13/50	35/50	
3	2	12/50	42/50	
4	1	8/50	18/50	
5	1	0/75	48/75	
6	1	24/75	63/75	
Total	9	53/325	222/325	$P < 0.00005$

* Number of gammarids eaten/number available.

the bottom, are negatively phototactic and which dive to the bottom when disturbed. The conspicuousness of the infected gammarid is increased further by the parasite's orange colour, which is visible through the integument of the host.

BEHAVIOUR OF PARASITES WITHIN THEIR HOSTS

The behaviour of the parasite itself may be an important feature of successful transfer even when it has no effects upon its host. The release of eggs is seldom a continuous process, but may occur only at times when the probability of encountering the next host is high. *Schistosoma haematobium* eggs are passed out of the body through the urine, and the majority are released at mid-day when, in a tropical climate, the probability of humans entering water is highest. *Enterobius vermicularis,* the human pinworm, by contrast, releases most of its eggs at night through the rectum in order to avoid faecal contamination and so to permit the eggs to disperse by air currents. The newly laid eggs are sticky, adhere to the skin and cause intense itching in children. The resulting scratching and lodgement of eggs under finger nails will also assist their passage to the mouth.

The release of cercariae is also often restricted to precise periods, especially amongst the schistosomes. Those of *S. bovis* are released at all times of day, but those of *S. mansoni* are generally released around mid-day when men enter water. Rodent strains of *S. japonicum* release their cercariae at dusk, when rodent activity is greatest. The eggs of monogeneans may also show periodicity of hatching. Those of *Entobdella soleae* hatch soon after dawn (Kearn, 1973). At this time the nocturnally active sole has adopted its diurnal posture of lying stationary and partly buried in the sea bed. There is thus a much greater chance of the slow moving oncomiracidium encountering a faster moving fish if it emerges in the daytime when the fish is inactive. By hatching at dawn, as opposed to a later hour, the larvae have the whole of the daylight period in which to contact their host. The ability of host mucus to enhance the hatch (p. 18) will enable some eggs to hatch at night should a sole come to rest in their vicinity.

Some species of *Plasmodium* also show circadian rhythms in activity (Worms, 1972). The gametocysts of *P. knowlesi* are mature and infective to mosquitos for a short period only (6–14 hours), and the cycle of asexual multiplication is adapted to ensure that this infective phase coincides with the time at which the vectors suck blood. The periodicity of microfilariae in blood (p. 50) is also timed so that maximum numbers are in the peripheral blood when the vectors bite. Thus the behaviour of parasites not only increases the probability of infection, but of infection by particular species.

SYNCHRONISATION OF HOST AND PARASITE LIFE CYCLES

For many parasites the probability of encountering a new host may be very low if the host itself is scarce or widely distributed, and infection may only be possible in practice when the hosts aggregate for a short period, as for breeding. It may also be necessary specifically to locate individuals of a new generation of hosts.

The life cycle of such parasites is therefore often synchronised with that of their hosts so that infective larvae are only produced or released when the hosts aggregate or when their progeny appear. This synchronisation may be accomplished by a common response to a climatic factor, or by reproduction of the parasite being related to and controlled directly by that of the host.

The ciliate protozoans *Opalina ranarum* and *Nyctotherus cordiformis* both have reproductive cycles synchronised with those of their host, the frog. In both cases control is effected by the sexual hormones of the frog stimulating reproduction of the parasite as well (p. 90). Another parasite of frogs, *Polystomum integerrimum*, a monogenean, behaves in a similar manner. Its genitalia mature as the frog prepares to enter water for breeding, and eggs are only produced when the frogs are in water and copulating, during a period of about one week. The time taken for the eggs to hatch corresponds to that required for frog eggs to develop into tadpoles at the internal gill stage, so that infective oncomiracidia and infective hosts are present in the same place at the same time. The parasite reproductive cycle in this case is controlled by the pituitary hormones of the frog.

The sporozoan *Leucocytozoon simondi* has a sexual phase synchronised with that of its host, the duck. During autumn and winter the level of infection within the adult duck is very low, but when the bird begins to mature and lay eggs in spring the level of infection rises, and is characterised by a high proportion of gametocytes. This ensures both that the infective stages are available when the vector, *Simulium*, emerges from its overwintering pupal stage, and that infective *Simulium* are in turn available at the same time as the young susceptible ducklings. By experimentally inducing earlier egg laying in the host it is also possible to induce a synchronous rise in gametocytes. This confirms the host control of the parasite cycle, but the exact mechanism of control is not known (Chernin, 1952).

The maturation of the rabbit flea, *Spilopsyllus cuniculi,* is also related closely to that of its host (Rothschild and Ford, 1964). The maturation of the ovaries of the female fleas occurs only after feeding on a pregnant female rabbit since it is stimulated and sustained by the rabbit's pituitary hormones present in the bood. After parturition, the fleas leave the does and live in the nest with the young rabbits, when they lay their eggs. Accelerated defaecation during flea maturation ensure faeces are available in the nesting material for the young fleas to feed on when they hatch.

Many species of monogeneans have cycles closely related to those of their hosts. *Dactylogyrus vastator,* a parasite of carp, begins reproduction in spring. This rises to a peak during summer, when the fish shoal for spawning and large shoals of susceptible juveniles are available. Several generations of the parasite may occur in summer (Fig. 4), but in autumn egg production ceases, and only a few parasites remain on their hosts. The mechanism of co-ordination is unknown, but is probably a common response by both host and parasite to climatic factors such as temperature and day length. The reproductive period of *Mazocraes alosae* is even more restricted. This species lives on the gills of shad, an anadromous migratory fish. For most of the year adults are dispersed

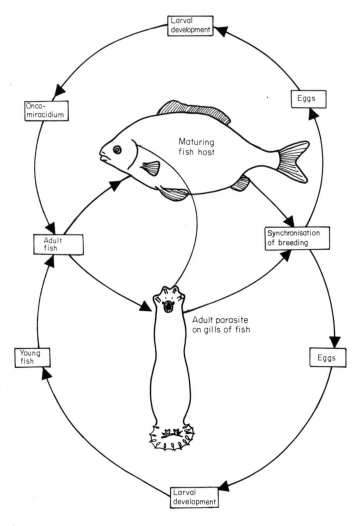

Fig. 4 The life cycle of *Dactylogyrus vastator*.

throughout the sea, and so are the young shad, but there is not any contact between the young and the old fish. In May, when adults mass off the estuaries prior to their upstream spawning migration, *M. alosae* produces eggs. These develop and hatch out rapidly, and reproduction and infection is confined to this month. For the parasite this is the only opportunity in the whole of the host's life history for infection to take place, whether of individuals of the same or of the new generation, and even the latter cannot become infected until they are old enough to start spawning. It must be presumed that the life cycles of the many other species of parasite of solitary marine fish are synchronised with those of their hosts in a similar way.

The life histories of many sheep nematodes are related to those of their hosts, but the situation is far more complex and involves changes in generation time, in rate of egg production and in host responses. In early spring, the new lambs are susceptible to nematodes such as *Haemonchus contortus*. They thus acquire infections, the eggs produced by the parasites contaminate the pastures, and they become re-infected. The cycle of re-infection continues throughout the summer; with increasing temperature the generation time of the parasites becomes shorter (Table 3), and the population increases exponentially (Fig. 30). About September the increase stops, as the immune response by the host becomes manifest, and the rate of egg production falls to a level comparable to that in adult sheep. Larvae infecting at this time are inhibited in their development, do not become adult, and remain in an inactive state within the sheep. Most of the eggs produced die since they are unable to survive the winter conditions, and the parasite overwinters within the sheep. The following spring, after parturition, the immune response of the sheep declines, as a direct consequence of its reproductive cycle. This removes the feedback control that had inhibited the development of the inactive larvae, and these now mature, producing a spring or post-parturient rise in egg production (Fig. 30). By the time these eggs have produced infective larvae the adult sheep have resumed their normal immune state, but the susceptible proportion of the host population has been enlarged by the appearance of the lambs, and the whole cycle re-commences. The post-parturient rise is thus not only the final feature in a series of events concerned with the transmission of parasites from one host generation to another but also the key feature in the timing of the whole series (Crofton, 1963). It is directly under the control of the host's immune system, which is in turn influenced by the host's reproductive cycle.

3 Specificity

GENERAL CONSIDERATIONS

Whatever method of dispersal is adopted and whatever the mechanism of host location, the infective stages of a parasite are likely to make contact with several potential host species, either by encountering them in the course of their random movements or by being ingested by them. Some of these will be the parasite's preferred or normal host species, with which it will establish a balanced, stable host-parasite system. Others, however, will be uncommon or abnormal hosts, with which the parasite will be unable to form any system at all or only an unstable one. Parasites forming systems with only one or a very few host species are referred to as being very host specific.

Although it might be expected that all parasites will be able to form a range of systems varying in their stability, this is not the case, as specificity varies widely between different species of parasite. Some are very narrowly specific, often to a single host species, and unless other factors in their life cycle ensure that they only contact the correct host species they will experience heavy mortality as a result of infecting other species. The majority of parasites, however, are less specific and are able to form stable systems with more than one host species and systems of varying stability with others. These will also experience some mortality as a result of infecting the wrong hosts, and in addition growth and reproductive rates may be reduced in unstable systems.

A comparable, though not parallel, situation exists amongst free living animals: most species are able to live in a range of habitats, but some are optimal and some barely tolerable. In these latter habitats both growth and reproduction of the species may be severely affected. Some species, however, have very restricted requirements, and can survive in only a single type of habitat. Specificity differs from this in that both the host and parasite and their mutual reactions are involved in the establishment of a host-parasite system, but it clearly has a profound influence upon both the distribution and abundance of a parasite.

ESTABLISHMENT OF HOST-PARASITE SYSTEMS

There are three essential requirements for the establishment of a host-parasite system. In the first instance the host and parasite must make contact with each other. The extent to which they do so depends upon their dispersal methods and their behaviour, and upon the ecological conditions prevailing in the habitat.

The second requirement is that the host must provide suitable conditions for the further development of the parasite. These conditions may be anatomical or physiological, but they are an innate property of the host which renders it suitable or unsuitable for the parasite. If the parasite has very restricted requirements its host range will also be very restricted, regardless of the frequency of contact with other species.

The third requirement is that the parasite must be able to withstand any responses of the host directed specifically against it. Virtually all animals react against invaders, whether by encapsulation, by phagocytosis or by production of antibodies, and the parasite must either avoid provoking this response or avoid its effects.

Only when these three requirements are met is it possible for a stable host-parasite system to exist, but none of them is necessarily constant and any or all may change with age, season, or climate. Changes in range or habitat of an animal may lead to changes in the probability of contact, as may aggregations of a temporary nature for purposes of breeding. The suitability of young animals may also differ from that of older ones, either because of differences in diet or in powers of resistance. In any host population, the susceptibility of individual hosts will also differ as a result of differences in physiology or responsiveness. Specificity is therefore not constant and static but must be considered a dynamic phenomenon.

PHYLOGENETIC ASPECTS

HOSTS RELATED PHYLOGENETICALLY

An examination of the specificity and distribution of parasites reveals that related species and genera of parasites are often restricted to related species and genera of hosts. In extreme cases the parasite is monospecific and only infects a single host species. The evident interpretation of this situation is that the host and parasite have evolved together and speciated together, and the relationship is therefore an old one. If this evolution has proceeded in a series of steps involving diminishing responsiveness on the part of the host and culminating in the recognition of the parasite as 'self', as Sprent (1962) has suggested, then evolution of such a system must have taken a long time, and stable systems, such as most monospecific systems are, must necessarily be old ones. Narrow specificity is therefore generally held to indicate an old system, and to reflect the phylogeny of both host and parasite.

Many parasites are indeed very specific, and especially the sporozoan protozoans including the species of *Plasmodium* and *Eimeria*. The Monogenea also show very narrow specificity. About 75% of the species infect only a single host species, whilst 95% are restricted to a single genus or family of hosts (Llewellyn, 1957). Genera of parasites tend to be restricted to genera of hosts, and within the large genus *Dactylogyrus* species only occur on more than one host when the hosts themselves are able to hybridise. Each order of birds has its own species of cestode, and the parallelism between evolution of bird cestodes and birds is very close (Baer, 1957). Even birds such as grebes and loons, with similar ecology, have different cestodes. In fact, the whole evolution of cestodes is closely related to that of their hosts. The orders Trypanorhyncha and Tetraphyllidea are confined to elasmobranch fish; Caryophyllidea, Pseudophyllidea and Proteocephala to teleosts, amphibia and reptiles, and a few birds or mammals with aquatic associations, and Cyclophyllidea to birds and mammals.

ENDEMIC HOSTS

Narrow specificity may also be encountered amongst the parasites of endemic host species. Old lakes, such as Lake Baikal, contain numerous endemic species, and some of these in turn harbour specific endemic parasites. In a few cases parasites may show very narrow specificity, yet the hosts are apparently completely unrelated. Larvae of the acanthocephalan *Echinorhynchus salmonis* are found in the arthropods *Pontoporeia affinis* and *Pallasea quadrispinosa,* but not in other species of these genera. The only connection between them is that both species are euglacial relicts of the old Yoldian sea. In these cases narrow specificity is again associated with an old relationship, but the important feature is the host's isolation rather than just its phylogenetic position.

HOSTS WITH SIMILAR MODES OF LIFE

The implication of phylogenetic specificity is that where a parasite is not monospecific, its other hosts will nevertheless be closely related, since closely related species are more likely to have similar modes of life and hence provide similar conditions for the parasite. This is by no means necessarily the case, since species not closely related may still have similar modes of life. It may therefore be the way of life of a species that is important in determining whether it can serve as a host, and hosts may be ecologically rather than phylogenetically related. Amongst adult Digenea in particular the hosts are more often in fact animals with similar ecological requirements. Thus, *Fasciola hepatica* occurs in grazing herbivores, including cattle, sheep, rabbits and, rarely, humans because of the similarity of their feeding habits, and *Posthodiplostomum cuticola* occurs in both herons and egrets. Amongst fleas, the hosts may be animals with similar ways of life, or species using the same nest or burrow for any purpose, including predators.

In many cases it is not easy to distinguish these aspects, since hosts with an unusual or isolated way of life may also be very old and phylogenetically isolated. Sturgeons have been both phylogenetically and ecologically isolated for a long period, and the narrow specificity shown by their parasites, with 30 species of various groups being specific to *Acipenser,* may be a reflection of either. The way in which both phylogenetic relationships and ecological similarities in mode of life have influenced specificity is clearly seen in the tapeworm genus *Eubothrium* (Table 11). The genus contains 9 species, infecting fish of 6 different families. Each species is however fairly specific, to the level of genus or species of host. Where specificity is wider than this, as with *E. crassum,* the other hosts have a similar mode of life and diet. Even *E. crassum* probably comprises two races

Table 11 The natural occurrence of adult tapeworms of *Eubothrium*.

Parasite species	Host	Host Family	Habitat and behaviour	
E. parvum	Mallotus villosus	Osmeridae	Marine	resident
E. arcticum	Lycodes pallidus	Zoarchidae	Marine	resident
E. clupeonellae	Clupeonella delicatula	Clupeidae	Marine	resident
E. fragile	Alosa fallax	Clupeidae	M & FW	migratory
E. acipenserinum	Acipenser spp.	Acipenseridae	M & FW	migratory
E. oncorhynchi	Oncorhynchus spp.	Salmonidae	M & FW	migratory
E. crassum	Salmo spp.	Salmonidae	M & FW	migratory
	Coregonus spp.	Salmonidae	FW	resident
E. salvelini	Salvelinus spp.	Salmonidae	FW	resident
E. rugosum	Lota lota	Gadidae	FW	resident

Only the most important hosts are listed, and *spp.* indicates that the parasite occurs in several species.

(Kennedy, 1969a), a freshwater one more specific to trout and a marine one more specific to salmon. The common feature of the hosts is that they are either anadromous, have descended from an anadromous stock, or belong to a family with anadromous members, with the possible exception of the fish genus *Lycodes*.

DYNAMIC NATURE OF SPECIFICITY

Whilst there can be little doubt that there does exist a relationship in many cases between the age of a host-parasite system and the specificity of a parasite, the relationship is not necessarily a very precise one, and other factors such as the mode of life of the host are clearly important. The phylogenetic argument for narrow specificity as evidence of an old relationship is itself rather suspect, since it lacks independent evidence or verification and is not susceptible to proof. It may be possible to demonstrate from a fossil record that a host is old, but not that the parasite itself is.

A further weakness in this approach is that it takes too little account of the dynamic nature of specificity and of the possibility of transfers from one host to another in the course of evolution. Once a host-parasite system has come into existence there are a number of possible courses for its further evolution. The host and parasite may both remain as they are, not speciating any further; both host and parasite may speciate together; or the parasite may speciate, but not the host. These three courses will result in narrow specificity. The host may, however, speciate, but not the parasite which may infect the newly evolved host species; the parasite may retain its original host but under the influence of changing conditions spread to new ones in addition; or, it may abandon its old host in favour of new ones. That this can in fact happen is shown by the history of *Fasciola hepatica* in Australia. The parasite was introduced into the continent in very recent times with sheep. Its European intermediate host *Lymnea truncatula* was absent, so it infected instead the local species *L. tomentosa* to which it has become very specific (Table 16). Narrow specificity in this case is not indicative of an old relationship.

Furthermore, a phylogenetic approach to specificity does not reveal any information about the nature of specificity or the factors responsible for it. It may indicate the probable course of evolution of a host-parasite system, but reveals nothing of the conditions that maintain the relationship or the consequences of it for the parasite population. Specificity is capable of altering over both long and short periods of time, and of changing as habitat and ecological conditions change.

MANIFESTATIONS OF SPECIFICITY

The records of occurrence of any particular parasite species will generally reveal the identity of its preferred hosts. Most of the records will come from these species, and a few from others, so the first indication that the host is not a normal one is that the parasite is found in it far less often. This may indeed be the only manifestation of specificity under field conditions, but in addition the parasite may be found to be smaller, retarded in development, or unable to mature in some hosts (Table 12).

The specificity of parasites is often narrower in the field than in the laboratory as a result of lack of opportunity to infect certain hosts. Under natural conditions there may be no ecological contact between a parasite and a suitable host, but when these are brought together the parasite may be able to infest it and develop normally. *Diphyllobothrium dendriticum* as an adult cestode is found in several species of gulls, but in the laboratory it also develops in rats and mice. These latter species do not normally feed on fish, its second intermediate

Table 12 The occurrence of *Pomphorhynchus laevis* in fish of the River Avon. (From Hine and Kennedy, 1974.)

Fish species	No. examined	% infected	Maximum burden	Parasite size (mm)	Gravid female parasites
Leuciscus cephalus	26	100	364	23	frequent
Leuciscus leuciscus	377	78	96	14	rare
Rutilus rutilus	22	64	5	6	absent
Barbus barbus	2	100	101	16	frequent
Tinca tinca	3	0	—	—	—
Gobio gobio	9	56	2	4	absent
Nemacheilus barbatulus	10	80	2	4	absent
Esox lucius	2	50	1	5	absent
Perca fluviatilis	1	100	15	8	absent
Anguilla anguilla	12	16	3	6	absent
Salmo salar	14	79	9	15	rare
Salmo trutta	9	84	141	12	rare
Salmo gairdneri	6	56	59	14	rare
Thymallus thymallus	74	100	429	10	absent
Cottus gobio	10	20	23	5	absent
Gasterosteus aculeatus	3	66	1	5	absent

host, and so there is normally no natural contact between them and the parasite.

In other cases, especially where specificity is dependent upon host un-suitability or resistance, it may be just as narrow in the field as in the laboratory. Kearn (1967) has shown that *Entobdella soleae* is found only on the sole, *Solea solea,* to which the oncomiracidium is attracted (p. 19). The adults are also capable of transferring directly from one sole to another. Only under artificially crowded conditions in an aquarium tank will the larvae settle on any other species of fish (Fig. 5), and even then the majority perish on most species after a short time. When adults were artificially transferred to other species, they remained alive on other soleids and on pleuronectids for only 24 hours. On elasmobranch rays they survived for 2–6 days, the same time that they were able to live attached to a glass plate.

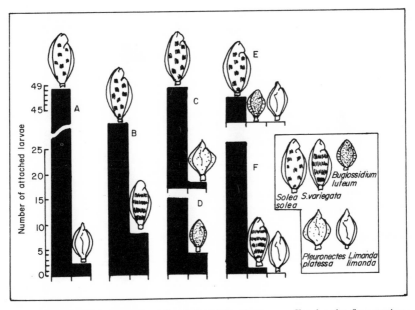

Fig. 5 Experiments in which oncomiracidia of *Entobdella soleae* were offered scales from various flatfishes, one of which was always *Solea solea*. The larvae were offered a choice of two sorts of scales (A-D) or three (E,F). (After Kearn, 1967.)

It is common, however, to find that parasites show a range of host-parasite systems in which they develop to different extents. Closely related species need not have similar ranges. *Schistosoma japonicum* shows little specificity towards vertebrates and can develop fully in a very wide range of species. *S. mansoni* can also develop in a wide range of hosts, but does not develop to maturity in some and may be capable of surviving for only very short periods in others. It can become fully mature in some 70 species of mammals belonging to 4 different orders, including the cotton rat and hamster, but in this last host it may cause considerable mortality. Albino rats, rabbits and pigs are susceptible to infection, but the parasite is not able to mature in them. Weasels are completely insusceptible. *S. haematobium* is far more specific than the other two species. Its natural hosts appear to be humans. Some species of monkeys and baboons can be infected, but the parasite may not mature in them. In both albino and cotton rats the numbers of parasites able to establish are reduced, and if eggs are produced they may not be viable.

Even where it is difficult to recognise the natural host in the field this may become clearer as a result of laboratory experiments. Procercoids of the tapeworm *Triaenophorus nodulosus* may be found in a variety of copepod hosts, but experimental infections show that these may be separated into five distinct groups (Table 13). The species in group V are obviously the preferred hosts, but those in group IV are nearly as suitable. Groups II and III can be regarded as accidental hosts. The parasites can survive in hosts from groups II–V, but the exacting requirements of the change from coracidium to procercoid are met by fewer species. The digenean *Paramphistomum microbothrium* occurs commonly in sheep, cattle and goats, but experimental infections reveal (Table 14) a very similar situation, with cattle clearly being the preferred hosts.

Table 13 Specificity of *Triaenophorus nodulosus*. (From Michaelow, 1955.)

Host group	Majority of larvae	Minority of larvae	Max. development
I	Digested in alimentary canal	—	Coracidia
II	Digested in alimentary canal	Penetrate to haemocoel	Coracidia
III	Penetrate to haemocoel	Develop to procercoids	Proceroids
IV	Penetrate to haemocoel—develop	Fail to develop	Procercoids
V	All penetrate haemocoel—develop	—	Proceroids

Table 14 Specificity of *Paramphistomum microbothrium*. (From Horak, 1971.)

	Sheep	Goat	Cattle
% infection 10 days	74.1	62	55
20 days	72.1	53	49
487 days	2.8	0.4	44
Pre-patent period	71 days	69 days	59 days
Egg production	declines	declines	persists high
Size	smallest	→	largest
Dose for acute fatality	40,000		160,000

The manifestation of specificity may also be dependent upon the age of the host. *Fasciola hepatica* is regarded as being specific to *Lymnea truncatula* in Europe and *L. tomentosa* in Australia. Experimental infections (Table 15) confirm this, but reveal also that it can infect the young specimens of other species. *L. peregra* can only be infected up to 3 days old, *L. palustris* to 7, and *L. stagnalis* to 14. When young specimens of these three species are infected, the initial establishment may be quite high, but then falls off when compared with the normal hosts, and very

Table 15 Experimental infections of *Limnea* with *Fasciola hepatica* from Germany. (From Boray, 1966.)

Species	Host Origin	Age (days)	Proportion of hosts with		
			Sporocysts	Rediae	Metacercariae
L. truncatula	Saxony	7–90	All	89–100%	All
L. stagnalis	Saxony	1–3	57%	10%	Few
		12–14	45%	Few	Few
		21+	None	None	None
L. palustris	Saxony	1–3	90%	72%	None
		7	50%	Some	Few
		56	None	None	None
L. peregra	Saxony	1–3	Some	Some	Some
		8–14	None	None	None
L. tomentosa	Australia	7–60	Most	Most	Most
L. lessoni	Australia	1–28	Some	None	None

few metacercariae are produced. With slightly older snails development is halted earlier, at the redial or sporocyst stage. Transplants confirm these results. Young rediae taken from young *L. stagnalis* and injected into older ones are killed within 7 days. In the preferred hosts, age of host has no influence upon the course of infection (Boray, 1966).

STRAINS OF PARASITE AND HOST

Even when it is possible to recognise clearly the preferred host of a parasite it does not necessarily follow that all populations of that host are equally susceptible to infection. Strains of both parasite and host, differing respectively in infectivity and suitability, have long been known to exist within each species. Parasites in particular by virtue of their self-fertilisation, polyembryony, asexual reproduction, clone formation and isolation are especially well suited to strain formation. Field investigations into the transmission of parasites and their epidemiology frequently produce evidence of the heterogeneity of both host and parasite populations.

Onchocerca volvulus, the nematode causing onchocerciasis or river-blindness, is widely distributed in tropical regions and is transmitted by species of *Simulium* (Appendix). The infectivity to the vector, to chimpanzees, its epidemiology and the symptoms of disease in humans differ between forms coming from the forest and savannah regions of West Africa, between forms from West and East Africa, and between forms from Africa and America (Duke, 1971: Nelson, 1970). Similarly, only some strains of the vector, *S. damnosum,* are anthropophilic and capable of transmitting the parasite, and these strains may become relatively more abundant following human settlement in an area. The local vectors are generally adapted to the local strain of the parasite in each region, and form more efficient hosts than strains from other regions.

Within a small area, strains may create separate host-parasite complexes. Within a single rain forest in the British Cameroons *Loa loa* occurs in both man and monkeys. The simian strain uses canopy dwelling species of *Chrysops* as vectors. The microfilariae show nocturnal periodicity, and the vectors bite when the monkeys congregate for the night. The human strain uses a different vector, one living in the lower regions of the forest and with diurnal biting activity, and its microfilariae show diurnal periodicity (Duke and Wijers, 1958: Duke, 1972). The human strain can be transmitted experimentally to mandrills, when it retains its diurnal periodicity, but under natural conditions this would rarely take place due to the behaviour of the strain and the ecological isolation of the vectors. Thus in the same area two strains are forming distinct host-parasite systems which exhibit different characteristics and rarely, if ever, interchange.

The breed and strain of bird host is also important in respect of susceptibility to infections of the protozoan *Eimeria*. Each species of the parasite contains several strains, and the result is a very narrowly specific relationship and a number of host-parasite systems with different characteristics (Horton-Smith and Long, 1963). Amongst the species of *Anopheles* that transmit malaria some races are much more suitable as vectors than others, and the parasites themselves comprise a number of strains. Resistance of *Culex pipiens* to *Plasmodium cathemerium* is known to involve races and to be genetically based (Huff, 1929). On feeding the parasite to the mosquito, development to the oocyst stage occurs in only about 50% of the insects. By breeding from eggs from resistant and susceptible individuals it has proved possible to produce susceptible strains in which 65% of the insects permit development and resistant ones in which only 7% permit it. The character responsible appears to be controlled by a single gene. In general susceptibility of *Culex* and *Aedes* species and races to *Plasmodium* appears to be genetically controlled (Garnham, 1964).

Compatibility of host and parasite strains is essential for the development of many cestodes and acanthocephalans, but strain specificity has been particularly studied amongst larval digeneans. Schistosomes have proved particularly interesting (Berrie, 1970; Wright, 1971). Miracidia of *S. mansoni* from Puerto Rica penetrate snails of *Biomphalaria glabrata* from Puerto Rica and Brasil with equal ease. In the Brasilian snails they provoke a cellular and fibrous tissue response which, together with phagocytosis, kills them within 24–48 hours, and none develop to cercariae. In Puerto Rican snails there is no tissue response, and cercariae develop in 95% of them. Progeny of crosses between snails from these two regions show cellular responses characteristic of each parent group and responses of an intermediate nature. The Puerto Rican hosts are also susceptible to Venezuelan strains of the parasite, but only 9% of them can be infected by an Egyptian strain. The Brasilian strains of snail are susceptible to Brasilian strains of parasite, but not to Puerto Rican, Venezuelan or Egyptian strains. In general it appears that larval schistosomes are infective to snails from their own endemic area, but not to those from other areas. The Japanese strain of *S. japonicum* is capable of infecting man, but although cercariae of the Formosan strain penetrate them, man and some other primates are resistant to infection and the parasites of this strain develop no further.

Fasciola hepatica also shows some strain specificity towards its intermediate hosts (Boray, 1966, 1969). Whereas *Lymnea truncatula* from Germany and Australia are equally susceptible to infections by European *F. hepatica* (Table 16), *L. tomentosa* behaves differently. It is far more susceptible to Australian parasites, which cause less mortality, than to German ones. More of the latter develop in unusual sites, and fewer survive to the redial stage.

Table 16 Experimental infections of the natural snail hosts of *Fasciola hepatica*. (From Boray, 1966.)

Host		Parasite Origin	Proportion with rediae	Host mortality	Larvae in unusual site	Minimum development time in days
Species	Origin					
L. truncatula	Germany	Germany	100%	17%	—	35
	Australia	Germany	100%	34%	—	35
L. tomentosa	Australia*	Australia	90%	49%	17%	28
	Australia*	Germany	65%	93%	53%	29
	Australia**	Australia	100%	25%	6%	29
	Australia**	Germany	90%	21%	27%	29

* 1st passage.
** 2nd passage.

The majority of parasites, and probably also of hosts, seem capable of strain formation, and compatibility is essential to ensure the establishment of a host-parasite system. Specificity may therefore be even stricter than appears at first, since the existence of strains is frequently only revealed by extensive laboratory investigations. Even monospecific parasites may contain a variety of host-parasite complexes, and the wider specificity of other parasites may well be more apparent than real. It would seem possible that in such cases there may exist several strains of parasite, each specific to a particular host. This would suggest that narrow specificity, at the strain level, may be more common even than appears.

FACTORS RESPONSIBLE FOR SPECIFICITY

ECOLOGICAL FACTORS

There is no single factor generally responsible for specificity. Numerous and diverse factors are involved, and their relative importance varies from system to system. Their actual identity is known in very few cases, since the detailed requirements of most parasites are also unknown. It is therefore very difficult to generalise about the causes of specificity.

For infection to take place at all, the host and parasite must obviously come into contact with each other. Under natural conditions the parasite may encounter only a very limited range of its possible hosts, and specificity appears narrower than it really is. To that extent the physico-chemical features of the habitat and the ecology of the host, factors which determine the possibility of contact, may be considered to influence specificity. Under the same conditions, however, the dispersal stages of the parasites also encounter a number of species that cannot serve as hosts. Although the behaviour of the parasite may ensure that only a small part of the population is thus wasted, infective stages, with a few exceptions, are seldom of real importance in determining specificity. This usually occurs after contact has been made. Conditions in the habitat only increase the probability of contact with a suitable host; they seldom confer selectivity upon the parasite.

This is well illustrated by the distribution of digenean larvae on rocky shores. James (1971) has shown that digeneans without free-swimming larvae occur in the supra-littoral fringe, those with two free-swimming larvae, i.e. both miracidia and cercariae tend to occur near lower tide level on more sheltered shores, and those with one free-swimming larva, the cercaria, are more widely distributed. This would suggest that the species in the supra-littoral fringe may be less specific, since they cannot select their hosts, than those with free-swimming larvae which are equipped with elaborate sense organs. A study of the host lists, however, fails to support this suggestion.

Laboratory investigations were able to clarify the situation to some extent. *Podocotyle atomon,* with two swimming larval stages, still showed little or no selection by cercariae for attachment to their intermediate host. Only amphipods, however, contained encysted metacercariae: cercariae, though attaching, failed to penetrate molluscs or crabs and degenerated on entering shrimps or fish. *Microphallus similis* was the most specific of all the species studied, being restricted to one species of crab, yet the cercaria was the least selective with respect to attachment to the intermediate host. Development to the metacercarial stage, however, could only take place in its preferred host, and cercariae entering other hosts were destroyed. By contrast, the conditions for the excystment of the metacercariae could be provided by a variety of birds as well as by rats and mice. Specific stimuli appeared to be unnecessary for the excystment of *M. pygmaeus* metacercariae also.

James concluded, therefore, that whilst ecological conditions such as the susceptibility of miracidia to desiccation were responsible for restricting the species with free-swimming larvae to the lower shore, host selection by free-swimming cercariae does not appear to contribute greatly to their specificity to their intermediate hosts. The host responses were far more important amongst the invertebrates, and the role of the cercariae was largely that of dispersal. In the vertebrate hosts, by contrast, specificity appeared to be related mainly to the diet and feeding behaviour of the bird.

BARRIERS TO PENETRATION

Immediately subsequent to contact, larvae have to settle on or penetrate their hosts. Whereas the miracidia of *F. hepatica* and most schistosomes penetrate nearly all the hosts with which they come into contact, the cercariae of schistosomes do not (Wright, 1971). The miracidia of *S. mansoni* are immobilised by tissue extracts of some abnormal hosts (Wright, 1966a,b, and p.   ), but in unsuitable hosts or strains they are generally destroyed after entry. Cercariae by contrast are often destroyed during the actual process of infection. The skin forms a major barrier to infection, and whereas that of hamsters, a suitable host for *S. mansoni,* is easily penetrated, a large percentage die in attempting to penetrate the skin of unsuitable hosts such as rats and mice. Death occurs in the Malpighian layer within 10 minutes. The skin therefore not only provides a penetration stimulus to schistosomes (Table 9), but also forms a selective barrier to infection.

This is true of other schistosomes also. Up to 30% of the cercariae of *Australobilharzia terrigalensis* die penetrating budgerigars, but 80% when penetrating ducks. In rats, at least, the state of the ground substances, especially the acellular glycoprotein elements, is the important factor (Lewert and Mandlowitz, 1963). Young rats are more easily penetrated since these elements are then least resistant to the larval enzymes. Old members of a strain of rats showing juvenile skin elements are also easily penetrated, whilst hypophysectomised rats, which resemble old rats in their skin characteristics, are seldom penetrated.

In the infections of copepods by larval *Triaenophorus* discussed earlier (p. 32), both the alimentary canal and the haemocoel can be considered as barriers to infection.

UNSUITABLE CONDITIONS

Parasites entering vectors may be killed rapidly by the unsuitable conditions in the alimentary tract of the wrong species (Nelson, 1964). *Dirofilaria immitis* can infect species of *Anopheles* since blood clots very slowly in their intestines, but in species of *Aedes* the blood clots too fast to allow migration of the parasite into the haemocoel. If anti-coagulant is added, the species can serve as a suitable host. The composition and state of the peritrophic membrane of the vector may also prevent penetration by some species of trypanosomes, but in other cases the intestine, for unknown reasons, is unsuitable for the development of a particular species of parasite.

Parasites entering hosts as resting stages depend, as has been shown (p. 16), upon receiving the appropriate stimulus for resumption of development. These are very rarely such that they can only be supplied by the preferred host, and are seldom involved in determing specificity. The reducing conditions necessary for hatching of eggs or excystment of larvae can generally be supplied by several species of possible hosts. In a few cases, such as the requirement for a very high CO_2 concentration for exsheathment of *Haemonchus contortus* larvae and the lytic effect of herbivore bile upon the cuticle of *Echinococcus granulosus* (Smyth, 1962), the range of hosts may be restricted by the precision of the stimuli required, but even within this range there will be some hosts that are still unsuitable for further development.

Once on or within a host a parasite may be unable to develop further for a variety of reasons. Suitable nutritional requirements may be lacking, or the parasite may be unable to establish sufficiently intimate contact with the host's tissues, or the surrounding medium may contain elements toxic to the parasite. The attachment structures of many parasites, especially amongst the Monogenea (Llewellyn, 1957), tetraphyllidean cestodes (Williams, 1960) and some other groups, are elaborate and highly specialised, and may only be able to function correctly on a few structurally similar and hence closely related hosts. Where attachment is possible and secure, the parasite may still be unable to feed. Thus, the monogenean *Entobdella soleae* can be induced to attach to species other than soles, but when it does so its period of survival is no longer than that of individuals attached to a glass plate and allowed to starve to death (Kearn, 1967). The human louse *Pediculus humanus* can be placed upon many non-human hosts, but it generally starves through refusal to feed, or if it does feed the blood may be lethal to it. The nutritional needs of most parasites are, however, unknown, and it is not possible to say how far failure to satisfy them is responsible for specificity. Probably they are very important, but in the present state of knowledge they have to be considered as part of the general host unsuitability.

Toxic serum elements not produced specifically in response to the presence of a parasite are responsible for specificity in some cases. Serum of *Raia radiata* contains natural antibodies which are toxic to the cestode *Acanthobothrium quadripartitum,* whereas serum of *Raia naevus,* its natural host, does not (McVicar and Fletcher, 1970) (Fig. 6). Serum of cotton rats also contains natural antibodies to *Trypanosoma vivax.*

HOST RESPONSES

Immunological or cellular responses by unsuitable hosts are also instrumental in determining specificity. In its natural hosts parasites are treated as 'self', but in unusual ones they are recognised as 'non-self' and the host responds to them to the best of its ability (Sprent, 1962, 1969). The nature of the response depends upon the capability of the host. Invertebrates respond to the presence of parasites in their body cavity by attempting to phagocytise them or encapsulate them (Tripp, 1969). If the parasite is a habitual one it is treated as host tissue and the responses cease, but if it is an alien one it may be destroyed or encapsulated. This latter response is not necessarily harmful, as the resting stages of many parasites in their natural hosts are contained within a cyst or capsule partly of host origin, and may survive for considerable periods. In some cases a layer of host tissue over the parasite may be the mechanism whereby the parasite comes to be recognised as self (Crompton, 1970). It was considered at one time that invertebrates only responded to nonspecific parasites, but it is now clear that they respond to all but the response to specific ones ceases rapidly. All parasites in the body cavity of unsuitable invertebrates, however, are destroyed by the host's normal defence mechanisms which are employed specifically against them.

Amongst vertebrates, the presence of specific anti-parasite antibodies can often be demonstrated in the serum of unsuitable hosts, but this is not in itself evidence that they are effective against the parasite. The cestode *Hymenolepis*

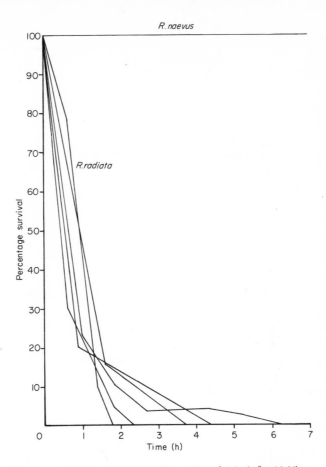

Fig. 6 The survival of *Acanthobothrium quadripartitum* in serum of two species of *Raja*. (After McVicar and Fletcher, 1970.)

microstoma induces antibody formation in its normal mice hosts (Moss, 1971), but not in rats, an abnormal host. Yet, in this abnormal host development ceases at about day 9 and the parasite sheds its proglottids and eventually dies and is shed from the host (Goodall, 1972). No serological reaction is detectable, drugs supressing the immune response do not affect the course of the infection, secondary infections can establish as easily as primary ones, and it can only be concluded that the conditions in the rat are generally unsuitable for the parasite and that an immune response is not involved.

By contrast, *H. diminuta* does not induce antibody production in its normal host the rat. In mice it grows normally until day 10, when it starts to shed proglottids in some strains of host (Fig. 7). These parasites may persist in the host, but undergo no further development unless they are transplanted to a fresh host (Hopkins *et al.,* 1972). The establishment rate in secondary infections is reduced and worms grow at a slower rate. Drugs supressing the immune response permit normal development of the parasite. There seems little doubt

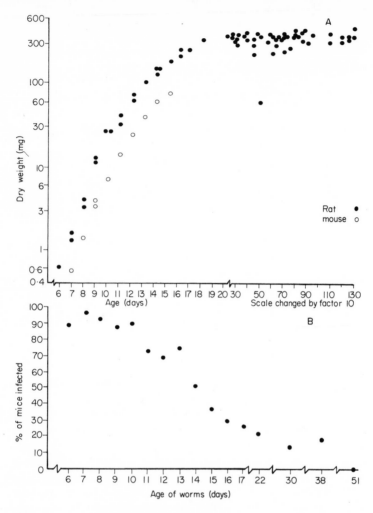

Fig. 7 A. A comparison of the growth rate of *Hymenolepis diminuta* in rats and mice. Destrobilated worms in mice are not included; B. A survivor-ship plot of *H. diminuta* in single worm infections in male mice. (Both after Hopkins et al., 1972.)

therefore that responses by mice to *H. diminuta* are immunologically mediated, but not those by rats to *H. microstoma*.

Specificity to plerocercoids of *Schistocephalus solidus* also appears to be immunologically controlled in some cases, but not in others. Procercoids are unable to infect the golden barb, since they are unable to penetrate the intestinal wall. They can, however, infect both the three and ten-spined stickleback. In the former species they develop normally, but in the latter growth is slower and has ceased between 6 and 8 days (Fig. 8). Death ensues between days 11 and 14 depending on temperature. After infections administered at days 14 and 28 to the three-spined stickleback, a third infection establishes (Orr *et al.,* 1969), but is

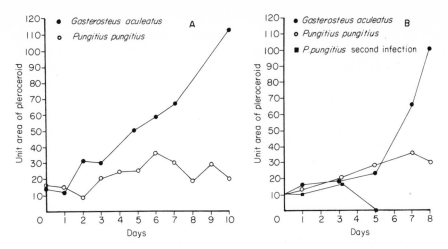

Fig. 8 The growth of *Schistocephalus solidus* plerocercoids in two species of sticklebacks. (After Orr *et al.*, 1969.)

rejected in the ten-spined stickleback in a faster time of 3 to 5 days. In this species the tegument of the parasite sustains severe damage at about day 8, but not in the three-spined stickleback. Transplants are possible and successful from one three-spined to another, but are killed in about 12 days in the ten-spined. It appears therefore that an immune response is involved in the failure of the parasite to establish in the ten-spined stickleback, but other fish are unsuitable hosts for other reasons.

Whilst therefore immune responses are undoubtedly involved in determining specificity of some parasites, it is very difficult to separate their role from that of other factors which render the host unsuitable, and in very few cases indeed has their effectiveness been unequivocably demonstrated. The behaviour of many parasites, especially nematodes, in unsuitable hosts shows close similarities to their behaviour in individuals of their normal species that have been immunised against them. Many of the manifestations of specificity including reduction of establishment, slower development and growth rates, stunting, suspended development and reduced reproductive rate are also indicative of an immune response. Whilst this may also suggest that immune responses are more often involved in specificity, it also indicates how difficult it is to show this conclusively.

BREAKDOWN OF SPECIFICITY

UNDER NATURAL CONDITIONS

In a stable ecosystem the factors responsible for determining specificity are generally themselves also stable, and specificity is strictly maintained. If, however, the ecosystem is altered, either naturally or as a result of human intervention, specificity may also alter. Parasites may establish new systems if brought into contact with new hosts, or the changes may favour its establishment in a host which is usually regarded as an occasional one. In this case the new host is frequently a species with similar ecological requirements to the usual host. *Azygia lucii* is a digenean fairly specific to pike, but perch, having a similar diet, is an occasional alternative host. In localities where pike are normally rare, or where their populations have suffered a heavy reduction for some reason, perch may become the normal host (Dogiel, 1961). The natural abundance of a host, because of its influence upon the probability of contact between parasite and host, is important to the maintenance of specificity under natural conditions. In Lake Ladoga, cyprinid fish are relatively rare, and the lake is dominated by salmonids. As a result the probability of cyprinid hosts encountering cyprinid parasites is low, whereas that of encountering salmonid parasites is high. As a result, cyprinids are frequently infected with salmonid parasites (Dogiel, 1961).

Under conditions of host stress, for example during the breeding season, host suitability may alter naturally, or its immune defences become temporarily less effective. This may permit the entry of unusual parasites, but the resulting system is generally unstable and of short duration since the return of normal conditions render the host unsuitable again.

AS A RESULT OF HUMAN INTERVENTION

Frequently the breakdown of specificity is a direct consequence of human intervention. The introduction of *Fasciola hepatica* into Australia has been discussed already (pp. 32, 35). In the absence of its natural host, *Lymnea truncatula,* from the continent it was able to infect the local species *L. tomentosa,* which occupies an almost identical ecological niche. Since then an Australian strain of the parasite has developed which can still infect *L. truncatula.* If the European strain is repeatedly passaged through *L. tomentosa* it can adapt to it, and a greater proportion of parasites develop to the redial stage at each passage (Table 16).

When Australian flukes are exposed to *L. peregra,* only young snails are susceptible and the minimum development time is 49 days. After one passage through *L. peregra,* the proportion of snails infected increases, older snails can be infected, and development time is reduced (Boray, 1966). Thus, under suitable field conditions such as the paucity of *L. tomentosa* or *L. truncatula,* the abundance of *L. peregra* and repeated exposure to this host, normal specificity could break down and *F. hepatica* could set up a new host-parasite system.

UNDER LABORATORY CONDITIONS

Many protozoans can adapt to new hosts under laboratory conditions. *Trypanosoma vivax,* a parasite of ungulates, is not able to infect rodents even if injected into them. When the parasite was injected into rats together with a quantity of sheep blood, then a few were able to survive and multiply (Desowitz, 1963). The essential requirement was the serum of the susceptible host, which altered the antibody activity in rats. The proportion surviving increased with each sub-passage from rat to rat, until after 37 sub-passages the parasite lost its dependence upon serum and could be transferred directly from rat to rat. Injection of cortisone, which supresses immunological responses, and the removal of the spleen enhanced the ability to develop in rats, and even then this was achieved more easily with some strains of parasite than with others. The adaptation was clearly complex, and involved loss of ability by the parasite to undergo cyclical transmission in its arthropod vector, alteration of virulence to its normal host, morphological, physiological and immunological changes in the parasite, and changes in drug sensitivity. Such a change is evidently not likely to occur or persist under natural conditions.

The selection and development of strains of parasites capable of infecting unusual hosts has now become a fairly common laboratory procedure, since many laboratory animals which are not natural hosts are far more suitable for experimental purposes than the normal hosts. Many parasites appear to have this ability to adapt to new hosts, and although it may not be evident under normal conditions, it can enable them to set up new host-parasite systems under changing conditions.

ECOLOGICAL CONSEQUENCES OF SPECIFICITY

Narrow specificity, enhanced by strain specificity, appears to be fairly widespread amongst parasites. This has undoubtedly arisen in many instances as a result of the host and parasite evolving and speciating together. By the time it has come to be accepted by the host as a normal parasite it must have acquired a number of adaptations that permit it to survive only under a restricted set of conditions, those provided by only a few species of hosts related phylogentically to the natural host or with similar ecological requirements. Similarly, the adaptations in the host necessary to enable it to tolerate one species of parasite will tend to prevent it from tolerating others. Such specialisation is of value to the establishment and survival of a host-parasite system, whilst simultaneously limiting the ability of both host and parasite to form new systems.

Such a situation would at first site appear to have certain disadvantages under natural conditions. Narrow specificity reduces the distribution of the parasite by restricting its host range, and may also decrease its abundance, since it may suffer mortality or reduced fertility in unsuitable hosts. The importance of this to the parasite population depends upon the extent to which encounters with unsuitable hosts take place within any particular locality. If this happens seldom, then narrow specificity is likely to be of little ecological consequence. If it happens often, then the situation depicted in Table 12 arises. In this locality a large part of the parasite population is located in unsuitable hosts, and although they survive, they are sterile and so contribute nothing to the next generation, and can be considered as effectively lost to the population. Narrow specificity is here responsible for considerable wastage. Thus, if a parasite shows narrow specificity and if a significant proportion of its population fails to locate its natural hosts, its mortality rate will rise and natality rate fall, with possible deleterious consequences.

In practice, however, such instances may be rarer than would at first appear, and in any locality the conditions tend to favour the natural host-parasite system. This suggestion is contrary to many widely held opinions, which are impressed with the apparent disadvantageous consequences of narrow specificity. However, the features of the life cycle that improve the probability of infection and especially the synchronisation of host and parasite life cycles increase the probability of contact with the correct host. The behaviour of the free-living infective stages also serves to increase the probability of contact, despite the frequent lack of specificity of the process. The identity of species used as intermediate hosts or vectors also increases the probability of the parasite being ingested or infecting the correct host. In any particular locality, the range of possible hosts is limited, and their behaviour in relation to that of the parasite's infective stages increases the probability of the natural hosts contacting the parasite. Where the parasite is ingested by hosts other than the preferred ones, its ability to form systems with alternative hosts does permit survival of part at least of the population. Even strain specificity operates in such a way that the hosts and parasites in any locality are compatible, and so places no restriction upon the distribution and abundance of the parasite. Finally, the ability of parasites to adapt to new hosts will also increase their chances of survival if conditions cease to favour their normal hosts. Thus, the ecological conditions prevailing in any particular locality tend to ensure that the deleterious consequences of narrow specificity to the parasite population are minimal.

4 Inter- and intra-specific relationships within a host

EMIGRATIONS AND SITE LOCATION

PREFERRED SITES

Virtually all parasites inhabit precise sites within or on a host, to the extent of preferring regions or parts of an organ to others. Crompton (1973) has reviewed the sites of intestinal helminths, and it is clear that in the majority of cases neither the reasons for the site chosen nor the method by which it is located are understood. Whereas blood parasites may circulate freely throughout the system, tissue ones may be much more closely restricted.

The behaviour of different species in one organ may vary. Amongst the species of *Eimeria* infecting chicken intestines, *E. brunetti*, *E. mivati* and *E. necatrix* sporocysts invade that part of the intestine in which they emerge from the oocysts, but if they do not hatch readily they will invade the caeca (Long, 1967). If *E. acervulina* and *E. maxima* are injected into the caecae, they not only fail to develop but also do not migrate to another part of the intestine. Sporocysts of *E. tenella* have a rigid site selection, since those hatched in the small intestine must proceed to the caecae before invasion. Even sporocysts of *E. praecox* find their way, by unknown means, to the small intestine after being injected into the caeca or cloaca.

Gill monogeneans are frequently restricted to particular gill arches (Table 17), despite entering the gill cavity in the general water current (Llewellyn, 1956). Some species such as *Diclidophora merlangi* show a distinct preference for one particular arch, whereas others such as *Axine belones* show only a tendency to occur less frequently upon some arches than upon others. In almost all cases the

Table 17 Distribution of parasites on the gill arches of some marine fish. (From Llewellyn, 1956.)

Host	Parasite	Total numbers of parasites per gill arch			
		1	2	3	4
Gadus merlangus	*Diclidophora merlangi*	53	8	1	4
G. luscus	*D. luscae*	7	118	91	8
Merluccius merluccius	*Anthocotyle merlucii*	4	28	7	5
Trigla cuculus	*Plectanocotyle gurnardi*	6	22	39	25
Trachurus trachurus	*Gastrocotyle trachuri*	41	56	46	20
	Pseudaxine trachuri	8	9	5	2
Belone belone	*Axine belones*	19	29	48	22

distribution is due to parasite selection, and cannot be explained in terms of water currents.

Nearly all intestinal parasites occupy characteristic regions of the alimentary tract (Fig. 9). Adult acanthocephalans and cestodes are generally confined to the regions specialised for the absorption of nutrients, typically the small intestine, and this is clearly associated with their need to take up nutrients over their body surface. Nematodes, by contrast, having an alimentary canal are able to feed in a variety of ways, and are accordingly able to occupy a much wider range of sites. Their small size also facilitates colonisation of nooks and crannies and of the intestinal wall itself, sites inaccessible to cestodes and acanthocephalans

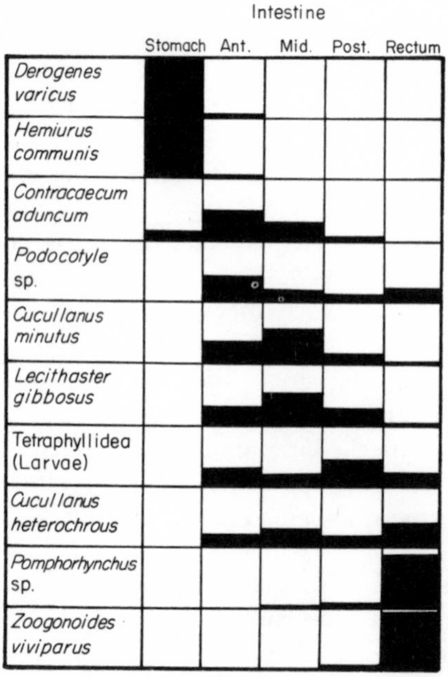

Intestine

	Stomach	Ant.	Mid.	Post.	Rectum
Derogenes varicus					
Hemiurus communis					
Contracaecum aduncum					
Podocotyle sp.					
Cucullanus minutus					
Lecithaster gibbosus					
Tetraphyllidea (Larvae)					
Cucullanus heterochrous					
Pomphorhynchus sp.					
Zoogonoides viviparus					

Fig. 9 Percentage distribution of parasites in the gut of flounders. (After MacKenzie and Gibson, 1970.)

Table 18 Mean position of *Schistocephalus solidus* in different hosts. (From McCaig and Hopkins, 1963.)

Host	Mean position (%) along intestine
Rat	74
Hamster	27
Duck	70
Chicken	53
Pigeon	30

(Crompton, 1973). Digeneans, despite their small size and the presence of a gut, occupy less varied sites. The site generally appears to be selected by the parasite. Adults and larvae of *Nippostrongylus brasiliensis*, a rat nematode (Appendix), occupy the anterior half of the small intestine, but if transplanted experimentally to other regions, are able to recognise that they are in the wrong region and migrate back to the correct ones (Alphey, 1970). The precise region may also vary between host species. *Schistocephalus solidus* can mature in several species of vertebrate, but the sites it occupies in each are not only different (Table 18) but are not even comparable in the conditions prevailing there.

MIXED SPECIES INFECTIONS

Where several species occur within the same organ, their distribution may be restricted by the presence of the other species. Eleven species of parasite were found in the intestine of flounders, but although the distribution of many of them overlapped to a greater or lesser extent (Fig. 9), the majority showed distinct preferences for particular regions. Within the stomach, *Derogenes* is commoner in the anterior region and *Hemiurus* in the posterior. In the intestine, tetraphyllidean larvae are found between the folds of the gut wall, whereas *Podocotyle* are found attached to the top of the gut wall (Mackenzie and Gibson, 1970). *Cucullanus heterochrous* is fairly evenly distributed throughout the gut for most of the year, but when *C. minutus* is also present in summer the majority are found in the rectum. Thus when both species are present they are restricted to separate regions of the gut. Whereas eight species of nematodes were found in the gut of *Testudo graeca*, niche diversification was evident (Schad, 1963), both linear and radial distributions of each species differed, and micro-habitat separation occurred. Indeed, differences in distribution of closely related species within the same organ are particularly common. In rats *Hymenolepis diminuta* occupies the anterior intestine, *H. nana* the posterior intestine and *H. microstoma* the bile duct.

EMIGRATIONS TO PREFERRED SITE

Some parasites reach their preferred site directly, especially protozoans such as trypanosomes and *Plasmodium* which are injected directly into the bloodstream. Others, however, undergo extensive migrations, often with accompanying mortality, either through the tissues or against a flow in the alimentary canal. The eggs of the nematode *Ascaris lumbricoides* are ingested by the definitive host and hatch out in the intestine, the site of the adult parasite, to release the second stage larva. Instead of remaining in the intestine, this migrates through the intestinal wall to the blood stream and passes via the hepatic portal system to the liver. From here they pass to the heart, and via the pulmonary artery to the lungs. They then moult twice, break into the alveoli, make their way up the trachea to the pharynx and thence to the small intestine.

The third stage infective larvae of *Dictyocaulus viviparus* also enter the host by ingestion, but before reaching the lungs, their definitive site, they pass through the intestinal wall to the lymphatic system, through the thoracic region and through the heart. Following a dose of 20,000 larvae, only 3151 were found in the lungs and 1082 in the lymph after 48 hours: a loss of almost 80%. The migration of *Trichinella spiralis* larvae in rats may involve a 47% mortality within 24 hours, and there is a loss during migration of *Nippostrongylus brasiliensis* larvae of between 40% and 60%.

The stimuli to migration have been studied in the larvae of the digenean *Diplostomum flexicaudum*. Metacercariae live in the lens of their host fish, and the parasites move to this site within hours of penetration. They die within 24 hours if they fail to locate the site, and they can enter any part of the body of the host (Ferguson, 1943). The larvae will penetrate eyes without lenses, although in reduced numbers. In fish with only a single eye, the parasites located in that eye and not in the empty orbit, so some part of the eye clearly provides the directional stimulus for migration. In this experiment they even travelled from one side of the fish to the other across the tissues in order to reach the single eye. When both eyes were removed, they were unable to localise. Cutting the optic nerve made little difference to location, but when the optic blood vessels were cut (Table 19) very few parasites entered the eye. Parasites were not attracted to lenses implanted in other parts of the body, so for this species the blood vessels of the eye appeared to provide the stimulus that enabled the parasites to locate their preferred site.

Table 19 Localisation of *Diplostomum flexicaudum* in experimental fish. (From Ferguson, 1943.)

Experiment	Status	No. of parasites/10 fish
Optic nerve cut in 1 eye	operated	264
	normal	3.75
Optic nerve + blood vessel cut in 1 eye	operated	1
	normal	740
Blood vessels cut in 1 eye	operated	4
	normal	565

Working with a similar species of parasite, Erasmus (1959) confirmed that entry could take place at any point on the body, yet the parasite would still localise in the eye. The migration took place through the connective tissue and muscle, not the blood stream (Table 20). Localisation was therefore again not due to chance migration, but to a directed movement.

Emigration may take place along the alimentary canal itself. Following ingestion and eversion of cysticercoids, *Hymenolepis diminuta* is swept along the intestine and attaches initially in the 30%–40% region of the gut. Between 7 and 10 days after infection, however, it moves foreward to attach in the 10%–20% region. Braten and Hopkins (1969) have demonstrated that if 7 day old specimens are transplanted to the duodenum, they return to the region from which they were moved and so they are evidently able to recognise and locate the

Table 20 The distribution of cercaria X following experimental infections. (From Erasmus, 1959.)

Time post infection	% of fish total in					
	Pharynx skin	Connective tissue	Blood	Nerves	Eye Wall	Eye Lens
15 minutes	84.2	0	0	0	0	0
55 minutes	19.5	59.0	3.1	0.75	0	0
5 hours 37 minutes	12.8	20.7	2.8	2.8	15.5	5.1
19 hours 6 minutes	3.4	3.4	3.4	0	0	72.6
139 hours 49 minutes	0	0	0	0	0	92.7

different regions of the intestine. By 18 days the scolex is still in the 10% region, but the parasite has grown to the extent of occupying almost 90% of the intestine. Throughout this period of growth the mid-point of the parasite remains in the same region. Since *H. diminuta* moves to a more posterior position in hosts whose bile duct has been cut it appears that the presence or concentration of bile is in some way related to the ability of the parasite to locate the preferred zone (Hopkins, 1970). The cestode *Raillietina cesticillus* by contrast moves with the flow of nutrients in the alimentary tract and migrates posteriorly from its initial position of attachment.

CHANGES OF SITE WITH AGE

In addition to the movements described above, some species change their site continuously with age. Oncomiracidia of *Entobdella soleae* are free swimming. Their host, the sole, spends a considerable time buried, except for the head region of the upper surface, in the sediment at the bottom of the sea. The larvae can therefore only infect in this region and post-oncomiracidia are restricted to it (Kearn, 1963). When the parasite reaches a length of between 1.0 and 1.5 mm it emigrates to the adjacent area of the lower surface of the fish (Fig. 10) where it remains for the rest of its life. The acanthocephalan *Echinorhynchus truttae* changes its position and moves down the intestine of its hosts all through its life (Awachie, 1966).

CIRCADIAN MOVEMENTS

The most sophisticated examples of rhythmical behaviour are found amongst the filarial nematodes. The microfilariae of these species circulate in the blood of their vertebrate host, and their appearance in the peripheral blood circulation exhibits a marked circadian periodicity (Hawking, 1968; Worms, 1972). Each species has its own intrinsic rhythm, dominated by host rhythms, which is related to the circadian rhythm of its vector's activity and ensures that the larvae are present in the peripheral blood at the time of the vector's greatest biting activity.

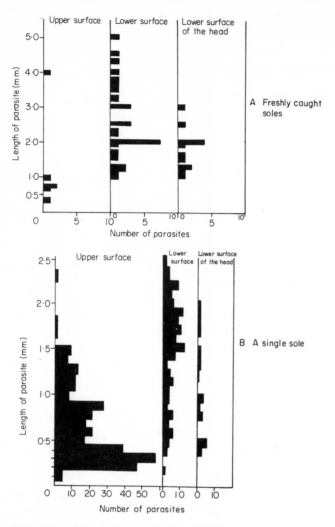

Fig. 10 The relationship between the lengths and numbers of *Entobdella soleae* on various parts of the skin of soles. (After Kearn, 1963.)

Wuchereria bancrofti microfilariae congregate in the small vessels of the lungs during the day, but at night, under the influence of changing oxygen tensions in the blood, they are evenly distributed throughout the peripheral circulation, reaching their maximum concentration between 2200 and 0400 hours. Their intermediate host is the night biting mosquito *Culex fatigans*. Human *Loa loa* by contrast shows diurnal periodicity (Fig. 11), again under the influence of changing oxygen tensions. The intermediate host in this case is the day biting *Chrysops silacea*. A strain of the same parasite in monkeys shows nocturnal periodicity (p. 34) in association with the nocturnal biting habits of the vector. *Dirofilaria immitis,* a parasite of carnivores, shows only partial periodicity, with the peaks in the peripheral blood at 0600 and 1800 hours, co-incident with the

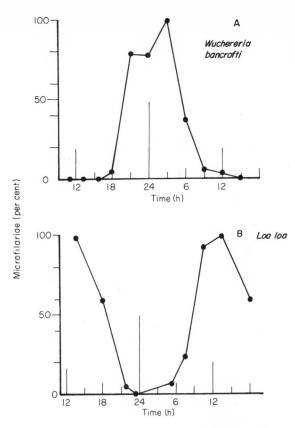

Fig. 11 Different patterns in the periodicity of occurrence of microfilariae in the peripheral blood. (After Hawking, 1968.)

two times of greatest biting activity of its mosquito host. *Litomosoides carinii* in cotton rats shows no circadian rhythm, but when the rats are quiet in their nests and their body temperatures fall, the microfilariae migrate to the peripheral circulation. At such times the mites which serve as intermediate hosts are more likely to bite.

The movements of *Hymenolepis diminuta* within the rat intestine also exhibit circadian rhythms in relation to the feeding regime of the host. In the experimental regime adopted by Bailey (1971), from about 1400 hours the quantity of nutrients reaching the rat intestine started increasing, reaching a peak at 2100 hours until dawn, and then diminishing until 1200 hours. Both movement and body length of the tapeworm were linked to this cycle. The body began shortening about 1500 hours, bringing the mass of the worm nearer to the inflow of nutrients. The worm began to extend again at 0600 hours, and at the same time the scolex moved foreward (Fig. 12). At this time the flow of nutrients had probably begun to decrease. When the stomach was almost empty, the scolex moved backwards, the body lengthened again, and it occupied the most rearward position about 1800 hours. Alterations in the host feeding

51

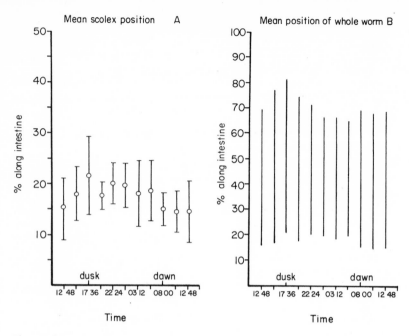

Fig. 12 The mean positions of *Hymenolepis diminuta* in rat intestines. (After Bailey, 1971.)

regime could alter the timing of the migrations, and in starved rats the scolex did not alter in position nor did the tapeworms exhibit periodic shortening.

EFFECT OF OTHER SPECIES ON SITE

The distribution of species in the same organ provides strong evidence (p. 47) for the importance of inter-specific competition, but conclusive evidence can only come from a comparison of the distribution of the species when they occur alone and together. *Hymenolepis diminuta* and the acanthocephalan *Moniliformis dubius* both occur in the anterior intestine of the rat. In concurrent infections Holmes (1961) found individuals of both species to be smaller than in single species infections. The tapeworm is more affected, and its growth is retarded to a degree proportional to the number of *M. dubius* present. When the two species are given to a rat simultaneously, both establish initially in their normal positions in the posterior intestine. After 10 days *H. diminuta* migrates anteriorly to establish in the 10%–20% region, again as normal. After three weeks *M. dubius* also moves anteriorly, to occupy the position of *H. diminuta,* which in turn moves backwards to settle behind the acanthocephalan and outside of its preferred region. If *H. diminuta* is given to rats already infected with *M. dubius*, it does not undergo its anterior migration at all. In hamsters, by contrast, the distribution of the two species is independent of each other, and competition does not apparently occur.

INTRA-SPECIFIC COMPETITION AND CROWDING EFFECTS

MANIFESTATIONS OF CROWDING

Once a parasite has reached its preferred site, it is likely to encounter individuals of its own species. As the parasite population increases, so does the pressure on the limited resources, leading to intra-specific competition. Competition is accentuated by the restriction of the parasites to a preferred site, and the effects made worse by the displacement of crowded populations to a less favoured site. This crowding effect is widespread amongst parasite populations, and is quite distinct in its causal mechanisms, though not in its manifestations, from host mediated immune responses.

Crowding effects are very evident in infections of birds with *Eimeria*. An increase in the infection dose of *E. praecox* leads to an increase in total oocyst production only up to a point, beyond which it starts to decline (Table 21). The reproductive index, however, falls consistently with increasing size of dose. The relationship is therefore not just a simple increase in the number of individuals produced in proportion to dosage. This is confirmed by a study of crowding in *E. tenella* (Table 22). 25,000 oocysts per bird appears to be the optimal dose, as

Table 21 Oocyst production in chicken infected with *Eimeria praecox*. (From Long, 1967.)

Dose given	4–5	5–6	6–7	7–8	Total	RI
	Oocyst production (m/bird)					
10^4	0.87	1.92	0.28	0.06	3.13	313
10^5	8.72	6.46	1.83	0.43	17.44	174
10^6	6.8	6.73	1.67	0.07	15.27	15

Days PI

RI = Number of oocysts produced/oocyst fed.

Table 22 Crowding in *Eimeria tenella*. (From Williams, 1973.)

Infection rate (oocysts/bird)	% mortality of birds	from faeces	from caeca	Total
		oocysts/bird in millions		
4,100,000	100	—	—	—
1,100,000	90	2.429	—	2.429
340,000	40	3.410	0.300	3.710
96,000	0	24.710	0.760	25.470
25,000	0	27.994	0.240	28.234
7,000	0	15.533	0	15.533
1,000	0	11.504	0	11.504
250	0	2.616	0	2.616
63	0	1.482	0	1.482
16	0	0.471	0	0.471

above this oocyst production declines, due in part to the formation of caecal cores, and in part to the destruction of the parasite's habitat by destruction and sloughing off of epithelial cells.

Nearly all species of cestodes appear to show crowding effects. At low densities the growth of *Hymenolepis microstoma* is slow at first, then rapid up to the nineteenth day, when it levels off. At high densities the percentage take falls slightly, but the mean weight of parasite tissue per mouse does not continue to rise but reaches a plateau, whilst the weight of individual parasites decreases in relation to the size of the infection (Fig. 13). Crowding effects do not become apparent in *H. diminuta* until about the seventh day after infection (Roberts, 1961). The size of the parasites decreases in proportion to the parasite burden, but although crowded worms are smaller, their surface area per unit weight is larger, suggesting that it is some resource passing in through the surface that is

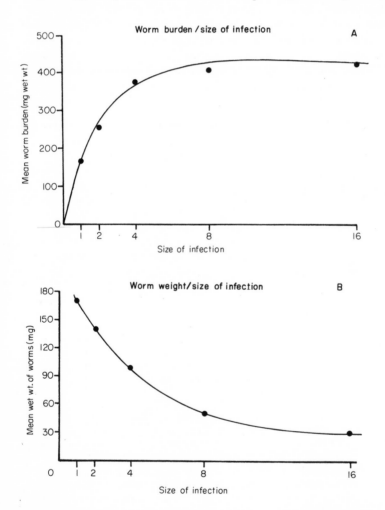

Fig. 13 The effect of crowding on *Hymenolepis microstoma* in mice. (After Moss, 1971.)

in short supply. The effect increases in the later growth stages as the worms become bigger. Maturation is never prevented, and its timing and rate appear to be unaffected by and independent of the growth rate. Nevertheless, the number of mature proglottids may be reduced and the number of gravid ones severely affected in crowded populations. All these effects are similar to those evidenced in starved hosts, and in the opinion of Roberts (1966) they are due to competition for carbohydrate resources. Recent work on some cestodes, however, has suggested that whilst the number of eggs produced per individual parasite may decline in crowded conditions, the number of eggs per host may be very much the same at all levels of infection and so the overall production is not decreased (Halvorsen and Andersen, 1974).

Crowding effects are known in other groups of parasites, and amongst nematodes and digeneans, establishment of the parasite is also frequently affected. The establishment and development of *Fasciola hepatica* in sheep can be severely affected by overcrowding (Table 23). In very heavy infections no parasites, or only a few, may become patent, and the pre-patent period, and so the generation time, is increased. Although the number of eggs per fluke declines, the number per sheep does not (Table 24) but continues to rise. It is possible that with this species some of the effects are due to liver fibrosis produced by heavy infections rendering the habitat less suitable for the flukes.

Table 23 Crowding of *Fasciola hepatica*. (From Boray, 1969.)

Infection dose	% established	Pre-patent period
200	51	56 days
500–1000	40	63 days
2000–10,000	35	13–15 weeks

Table 24 Egg production of *Fasciola hepatica*. (From Boray, 1969.)

Average no. of flukes	egg/fluke/day	egg/sheep/day
19	25,099	476,881
70	20,015	600,450
137	16,881	2,312,697
237	12,309	2,917,233
401	8,832	3,542,033

Within invertebrate hosts crowding effects are less common. Although the growth rate of many procercoid cestodes within copepods is often inversely proportional to the number of parasites present, there is no indication that overcrowding of digenean larvae in snails affects either their development or rate of cercarial production. Overcrowding of filariae in their vector appears often to be prevented by the failure of many larvae to leave the mid-gut and enter the haemocoel. Amongst invertebrates also overcrowding leads far more often to the death of the host.

CONSEQUENCES OF OVERCROWDING

Overcrowding, by reducing establishment, growth rate and egg production and by increasing generation time, can reduce the size of parasite populations. The most significant of these effects in this respect is probably the increase in generation time, since this will markedly decrease fecundity (p. 10). Intra-specific competition can therefore operate to limit the size of a parasite population in a manner directly comparable to the way in which it operates amongst free living animals. Since its effects increase in severity as the population increases in size, it can function as a negative feedback control and achieve a homeostatic system.

Wisniewski (1958) has suggested, indeed, that intra-specific competition is a major control upon parasite populations, and is certainly responsible for the size structure often found in tapeworm populations. The majority of parasites are stunted and checked in their development at high densities, and so are unable to harm the host. They are surviving almost in a latent state, but following death of any individuals the checks are removed and the parasites resume normal development.

On the other hand, if the numbers of eggs produced per host, as opposed to per parasite, are the same or increase with crowding as happens with *F. hepatica,* then the effectiveness of intra-specific competition as a feedback control must be reduced. This is to be expected ecologically, since hosts must frequently ingest large numbers of parasites simultaneously as a direct consequence of the over-dispersion of the parasite in its larval stages (p. 67). If there were always to be a heavy loss of individuals or eggs associated with crowding, then this could render overdispersion disadvantageous. Clearly in many animals there is an optimum density, and in others no crowding effects appear to operate. Whilst therefore intra-specific competition can act as an important feedback control upon parasite population size, it must not be assumed that it actually does so in all cases, or that it is equally effective in all host-parasite systems.

INTER-SPECIFIC RELATIONSHIPS

TYPES OF RELATIONSHIP

Although the different requirements of each parasite species and their different sites and micro-habitats generally prevent inter-specific competition for limited resources, the parasites may still come into contact with other species and be affected by them. Competition is only one of the possible interactions between species populations. In addition the species could actually interfere with each other in the course of their migrations or in their definitive sites, one species could damage another by eating it, or, most importantly, the presence of one species could induce a host response that would be effective against another or render the habitat less suitable for it.

Since, therefore, parasite species may inter-react for a variety of reasons, a variety of responses is possible. This variety makes generalisations and predictions about inter-specific relationships very difficult. Species may fail to inter-react because they inhabit different parts of an organ, or they may have a striking effect on each other through the mediation of host responses. It is equally difficult to predict whether any inter-reaction will be reciprocal or not. Most of the characteristic inter-reactions between free living animals can also occur between some parasite species, but the effect of one parasite population upon another is more often spasmodic, fortuitous and unpredictable.

COMPETITIVE INTER-REACTIONS

Inter-specific reactions can only be demonstrated conclusively by experimental procedures. Observation of natural populations may suggest that they occur, but correlations between the presence or absence of two species may have several causes. In a detailed study of the parasites of brown trout, Thomas (1964) showed that the majority of species were independent of, and had no effect upon, each other. Positive correlations were, however, observed between the presence of three pairs of species. These were not due to any interactions between the species, but arose because the ecological and habitat conditions favouring infection with one of the pair also favoured the other, and the infective larvae of each pair of species tended to occur in the same region of the river. Negative correlations were observed between three other pairs of species, which tended to occupy the same region of the alimentary tract. Whilst this exclusion suggests competition, it is also possible that if the host fish fed upon the invertebrate host of one species, its food preference would tend to exclude it from acquiring the hosts of the other.

Conclusions based on the analysis of field data must, therefore, always be accepted with caution, unless additional information is available. Thus the observation that *Haematoloechus* sp. and *Rhabdias bufonis* seldom occur together in the lungs of frogs suggests, but does not prove, competition, whereas the observation that *Phyllodistomum folium* rarely occurs together with *Myxidium lieberkuhni* in the bladder of pike coupled with the knowledge that the digenean can and does ingest the protozoan does suggest a direct interaction between the two species. Most often field observations fail to indicate any inter-relationships between parasite species. Most infected snails carry only a single species of larval digenean, but this may be due very often to the low probabilities of any miracidium infecting a snail, and the occasional occurrence of two or more species in one host individual suggests there is little or no inter-reaction between species. Similarly there appear to be no reactions between the species of microfilariae within their vectors, although concurrent infections are rare for ecological reasons.

Experimental confirmation of competition may also be difficult to obtain, as it is generally avoided by the restriction of each species to its favoured site (p. 47). It has, however, been demonstrated to occur between *Hymenolepis diminuta* and *Moniliformis dubius* (p. 52) and *H. microstoma* and *Fasciola hepatica* in the bile ducts of mice (Long, 1967). In single species infections each species lives in the proximal bile duct. Under one particular set of conditions 77% of the *F. hepatica* administered established, and the average weight of each parasite was 46 mg. The corresponding figures for *H. microstoma* were 80% and 428 mg. In concurrent infections, 88% of *F. hepatica* established, with a weight of 49 mg per fluke, whereas only 50% of the tapeworms established, with a weight of 250 mg, and then in the distal bile duct. These two species clearly compete in mixed infections, with the fluke being the more successful.

Simultaneous infection of *Gammarus pulex* by eggs of *Polymorphus minutus* and *Echninorhynchus truttae* results in both parasites growing at a slower rate than in single infections due to a general and non-specific crowding effect (Awachie, 1967). Neither species, however, confers resistance against the other or facilitates its infection and they do not appear to compete with each other in the generally accepted meaning of the term. It must be concluded therefore that inter-specific competition can occur and is usually detrimental to one or both species, but it is of fairly rare occurrence and of little significance in controlling the size of parasite populations.

PREDATION

Inter-specific predation has seldom been demonstrated, and would indeed be expected to be uncommon. Field observations, however, frequently indicate an antagonistic reaction between echinostomes and other groups of digeneans within a single snail (Lie *et al.*, 1965). This has been noted to occur especially between predatory echinostome rediae and *Fasciola* sporocysts, and between echinostomes and *Schistosoma mansoni* sporocysts. It has been shown that echinostomes prey directly upon sporocysts of schistosomes, strigeids and xiphidocercaria. Even between themselves some species of echinostomes dominated others. Infections of *Biomphalaria glabrata* with two species of echinostome revealed that *E. lindoense* was always destroyed, since it was unable to eat the rediae of the other species but was itself susceptible to predation. It did not survive even when given as the first infection, and attempts to infect snails already carrying the other species were rarely successful.

CROSS-IMMUNITY

Immunity induced by protozoan infections is generally very specific, and cross-immunity between species is not very common. Nine of the species of *Eimeria* infecting chickens induce selective and very specific responses. These are effective against the species inducing them but not against any other, and there is no cross-immunity. Some instances of cross-immunity are known, however (Table 25), and birds infected with *E. maxima* are almost immune to *E. brunetti* and vice versa. Whereas immunity induced by one strain of a species may not be effective against another strain, in some cases (Table 26) it can at least confer partial immunity upon the host.

Amongst the malarial parasites, cross immunity between species of

Table 25 Cross infection with *Eimeria* species. (From Rose, 1967.)

| | 1st infection immunising | |
	E. brunetti	E. maxima
No second infection	38.54	84.03
2nd infection challenge E. brunetti	0	0.11
E. maxima	8.3	0

Total faecal oocyst production after final infections as mean/m bird/group.

Table 26 Cross infection with *Eimeria acervulina* strains. (From Joyner, 1969.)

Expt.	A				B			
Immunising strain	Strain W		Control (Nil)		Strain M		Control (Nil)	
Challenge strain	W	M	W	M	W	M	W	M
Oocyst output (m per bird)	0	57.7	380.2	562.5	1.740	0	411.5	1086

Plasmodium is rare or completely absent (Garnham, 1970; Zuckerman, 1970). Although closely related species may share antigens in common, the resulting antibodies are usually specific in their action. A degree of cross-immunity does however occur between strains of *P. berghei,* and *P. vaughani* can confer some degree of protection on canaries against infections by other bird malarias (McGhee, 1970). Amongst the flagellates, *Leishmania tropica* can protect against *L. brasiliensis* and *L. mexicana,* and the strain of leishmaniasis characterised by the production of wet lesions can also confer some protection against the strain producing dry lesions (Stauber, 1970). Despite the extremely specific nature of the immune responses to trypanosomes some degree of cross-immunity is also possible between the strains of *T. cruzi,* and endo-antigens of *T. vivax* and *T. brucei* can elicit some cross-immunity.

It has been appreciated for some time that the self-cure induced by *Haemonchus contortus* could also eliminate other species of trichostrongyle nematodes, but the inter-relationships between the species are very complex (Turner *et al.,* 1962). In lambs *H. contortus* can eliminate *Ostertagia circumcincta* and *Trichostrongylus axei,* whilst self-cure induced by either of the latter two species can eliminate *H. contortus* and *T. colubriformis. H. contortus* establishes better in single species infections than in mixed infections with either *T. axei* or *O. circumcincta* or both species, and in mixed infections its egg production is reduced. In mixed infections of one or more of these three species *T. axei* is at the most only slightly infected by the presence of one or both of the others, *O.*

circumcincta is moderately affected by one or both of the others, and *H. contortus* is adversely affected by both species, but especially by *T. axei*. Interactions between other nematode species are relatively frequent, and often involve host immune reactions.

On other occasions, apparently unrelated species may confer protection against each other. Since antibodies are usually fairly specific this is rather surprising, as it would seem likely that they would only be effective against closely related species which could be expected to have fairly similar antigens. However, as Schad (1966), has pointed out, similar antigens could arise in widely different species by sheer chance. Furthermore, if parasites in any host species do share antigens with those of the host and indulge in molecular mimicry as Damian (1964) believes, then there will be antigen convergence between the parasite species in any one host, and antibodies produced against one species will be effective against another, regardless of their relationship. In these situations cross-reactions could be expected between the two species. Whilst such a situation may exist in theory, however, it has not been demonstrated in practice, and the work of Smithers and Terry (1969) casts doubt upon the existence of such molecular mimicry.

In many instances non-reciprocal reactions occur between two species, and Schad (1966) has suggested that one species may, by chance, have produced antigens which elicit little or no effect against itself, but produce a response which does effect a potential competitor. Such antigens would be selected for specifically because of their effect on another species and because they minimise competition. Explanations of this sort may be sought for such interactions as mice infected with trypanosomes showing increased resistance to schistosomes, and repeated infections of mice with schistosomes reducing the establishment of *Ascaris suum*.

ECOLOGICAL CONSEQUENCES OF INTER-SPECIFIC REACTIONS

It is clear that inter-specific reactions are fairly widespread but are unpredictable in their manifestations. They may affect growth or establishment of one or both species, but seldom to the same extent as intra-specific reactions. Nor do they necessarily operate in a feedback manner. Many demonstrations of inter-specific reactions have taken place under laboratory regimes, and it is clear from these that the subsequent course of the mixed infection may depend upon which species was first to infect the host, and the interval after this at which the second infection was administered. In other instances cross-reactions could only be demonstrated under conditions unlikely to be encountered in natural populations. Even when manifested, cross-resistance is frequently only partial. Although therefore inter-specific reactions do exist, it is doubtful whether they are of much real significance in reducing natural populations except in a few cases, and they probably do not constitute an important control upon parasite numbers.

5 Dispersion of parasites within a host-parasite system

Two basic types of host-parasite system can be recognised (Fig. 14). In the first type, parasites are able to escape from the host either by their own efforts, as do cercariae, or by the activities of the host, as do trypanosomes and microfilariae when ejected in the course of their vector's feeding, or in response to host reactions, by dropping off the surface of the host or passing out through its orifices. This type of system is characteristic of all definitive host-parasite systems, and of some intermediate host-parasite systems, and of all host-vector systems. In these latter two cases transfer of the parasite to the next host does not necessarily involve the death of the host or vector, and indeed such death would be disadvantageous since it would also terminate the life of the parasite. Continual release of the parasite from the host is possible, and may contribute towards a reduction in parasite numbers.

In the second type of system, transfer from one host to the next is accomplished by ingestion of the infected host. This type is characteristic of many intermediate host-parasite systems. As far as the parasite is concerned, this is a trapped system since it can only escape from it by the death of the host. No other form of release is possible, and it can happen on one occasion only. Since death of the intermediate host is essential for the successful completion of the cycle, it is advantageous for the parasite to kill it or render it more susceptible to predation in such a way that the probability of its being ingested by the next natural host is increased (Chapter 2).

It might be expected therefore that the two types of system will differ with respect to the temporal changes in the level of parasite infection and the factors controlling this (Fig. 14). In trapped systems there is a tendency for the infection level to rise continuously, as the time to which the host is exposed to infection increases, and this tendency is accentuated if the parasite is capable of asexual reproduction when heavy infections of an individual host may arise following an initial infection by a single parasite. In the other type of system, since continual release of parasites is possible, the numbers may fluctuate with time or even remain steady.

In general, the level of infection in any host individual depends upon the number of parasites infecting the host and the responses of the host to the infection, i.e. to changes in recruitment and mortality rates. Recruitment in turn depends basically upon the numbers and availability of parasites in the preceding stage of the life cycle, and this in turn depends upon the reproductive success of the previous generation and the parasite's behaviour with respect to the host. It will also, however, be heavily influenced by the behaviour and

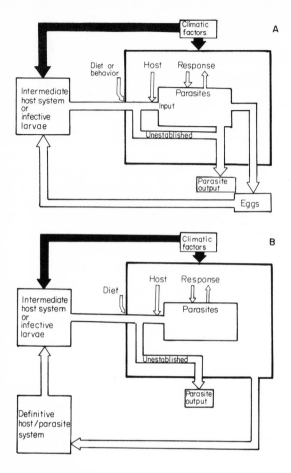

Fig. 14 Models showing the flow paths of parasites and some of the probable control factors in: A. a definitive host-parasite system; B. an intermediate host-parasite system in which the parasite is not released from the host except by death of the latter.

population density of the hosts. Mortality may be due to death during the course of the infection process, death as a result of a host response, and death at the natural termination of the life span. Some of the mortality factors in particular, such as host responses and intra-specific competition, are capable of acting as negative feedback controls and so stabilising the system.

All these factors can vary in time and space and the changes in each, in their relative importance and in their interactions will cause corresponding changes in the levels of infection within the host. Many of the factors are also influenced in turn by climatic changes, and when such changes are regular, the infection levels may change in a regular manner. The parasites in any host are thus at any time in a state of dynamic equilibrium, the level of which depends upon the rates of recruitment and mortality. This is true also for trapped systems, although the level here is dependent more upon recruitment. Since also the ecology of each individual host is different, then the infection level will differ and change in a different way in different individuals, and the infection is unlikely to be distributed in a uniform manner throughout the host population.

DISPERSION OF PARASITES THROUGHOUT A HOST POPULATION

IN RELATION TO AGE OF HOST

The older a host is, the longer it has had to make contact with a parasite. Thus, the incidence and the level of infection of many species of parasite change and increase with the age of the host. Change in age, however, often also means a change in structure, behaviour or diet, and so also a change in the probability of infection. Changes in host structure are responsible for changes in the infection of the protozoan *Myxosoma cerebralis*. This species is only able to infect cartilage, and so its incidence declines in older rainbow trout as ossification progresses. Similarly, parasites that live in the *bursa fabricii* of birds also decline in incidence with age of host. Due to difficulties in transmission, young mammals have very few endoparasites when in the suckling stage as placental transmission, though possible for some species of *Plasmodium,* is very difficult. By contrast, *Trypanosoma equiperdum* is transmitted during coitus, and so only occurs in mature animals.

Changes in the parasite fauna of a host with age have been studied extensively by Dogiel (1961), who suggested that in the majority of cases both the numbers and diversity of parasites increased with the age of the fish. Those parasites with a direct life cycle, especially protozoans, are the first to infect a host. In young (1 month old) perch, 4 out of 6 parasite species were protozoans, and of the other two one was a digenean with direct infecting cercariae. This situation is confirmed by a study of the parasites of pike (Table 27). Although *Acanthocephalus lucii* was independent of host age, the incidence of the majority of species and their level of infection increased with age of host. The decrease in incidence of *Proteocephalus percae* was associated with the change in the feeding behaviour of the host, which moves from a plankton to a fish diet and so no longer makes contact with the larval stages of this parasite. A similar situation is found within bird populations, and probably also amongst mammals although this has been studied less intensively.

The age of a host and its mode of life may be very closely inter-related, and it may often be the latter that determines the parasite fauna. Thus, lake trout frequently do not become infected with the monogenean *Discocotyle sagittata* until they are two years old, despite the parasite's direct life history. This is because the parasite infects fish in the deeper waters of the lake only (Paling, 1965), and trout do not move out of the nursery streams and into the lake until they are, on average, two years' old. Incidence and intensity of infection then rise steadily until fish are about five years' old, when they level off. By that time parasites have reached their natural life span of 3 years, and so although infection continues, the older parasites die as rapidly as the new ones infect and a state of equilibrium

Table 27 Changes in incidence and mean worm burden of some parasites of pike. (From Dogiel, 1961.)

Host age	Acanthocephalus lucii		Camallanus lacustris		Tylodelphys clavata		Tetraonchus monenteron		Myxidium lieberkuhni	Proteocephalus percae
	%	MWB	%	MWB	%	MWB	%	MWB	%	%
0+	35	2	6	1	53	35	47	2.8	23.5	70.6
1	7	1	20	1.3	59	7.4	87	15	100	26.4
2	33	1.2	20	3.6	80	26	87	23	100	13.2
3	13	1	26	2.7	86	75	93	54	100	6.6
4	15	1	29	4	88	44	100	56	100	14.7
5>	40	5.7	46	7.3	86	42	100	139	100	19.0

is reached. In natural habitats the monogenean *Dactylogyrus vastator* is found only on younger carp. This is not due to any resistance as such by the fish, since experimental infections of older fish can be achieved easily (Dogiel, 1961). The explanation lies in the fact that younger carp are surface dwellers and so are more likely to encounter the larval stages of the parasite, which remain in the surface waters, than are older carp which are bottom dwellers. In many cases the greater volume of food ingested by an animal as it becomes larger is sufficient explanation for the increase in the numbers of a parasite.

Where a host is able to respond immunologically to a parasite, then the pattern of increasing numbers of parasites with age may alter. In a population of rabbits in New Zealand, the incidence of *Taenia pisiformis* increased steadily with host age as the time of exposure to the parasite and hence probability of contact increased (Ball, 1964). The average level of infection, however, decreased as soon as the rabbits were old enough to exhibit an immune response, and then levelled off and remained steady. Most mammals are in fact more susceptible to infections in early life until their immune systems are fully developed.

IN RELATION TO BEHAVIOUR AND MOVEMENTS OF HOST

Many animals undergo marked changes in behaviour in the course of their life which are associated with changes in their parasite fauna. Carp aggregate in large numbers at the bottom of ponds for winter, when they feed little. They thus tend to lose their endoparasites, which are not replaced until the carp resume feeding in spring. The ectoparasitic leeches however tend to increase in numbers at this time since the behaviour of the fish, and in particular their aggregation and sluggishness, favour their transmission (Dogiel, 1961). Animals that aggregate in colonies for breeding purposes also tend to acquire larger numbers of ectoparasites at the same time, since the probability of contact between parasite and host increases for this short period. Mating is in fact the only time when birds such as cuckoos can acquire their specific parasites, since these cannot be obtained from their foster parents in the nest. Hibernation is also associated with changes in parasite fauna (Dogiel, 1964). In most cases the level of infection declines, since recruitment of parasites is difficult or impossible, especially for endoparasites. In some cases the parasites may develop as normal over this period, but in others they also enter a resting stage.

The parasite fauna of frogs also reflects closely the changes in the host's mode of life. Tadpoles are infected almost exclusively by ectoparasitic protozoans, although the monogenean *Polystoma integerrimum* occurs on the gills. At the time of metamorphosis the ectoparasitic protozoans disappear, and are replaced by endoparasitic ones such as *Opalina ranarum* and *Nyctotheres cordiformis*, which may even have appeared in the late tadpole stage. The metazoan fauna, including the characteristic flukes and nematodes, only appears after metamorphosis. During metamorphosis itself, *P. integerrimum* moves from the gills to the bladder (Dogiel, 1964).

Changes in parasite fauna are particularly evident in association with host migrations. Young salmon in the River Exe have a very similar fauna to that of trout, but it is reduced in diversity. The longer they stay in the river, the more diverse it becomes. This complete fauna is lost, however, when they migrate to the sea (Table 28). On their return from the sea they carry a fauna of marine parasites, and these are gradually lost or reduced in numbers during their journey up river. Some are lost almost immediately on entry to fresh water, especially the endoparasites, some decline slowly, and some, such as the encysted *Anisakis* larvae, are unaffected by fresh water.

Table 28 The incidence (%) of parasites in salmon of the River Exe, England.

Parasite species	Host species					
	Trout			Salmon		
		Parr	Smolts	Fresh adult	Spawning adult	Kelt
Discocotyle sagittata	P	0	0	0	0	0
Neoechinorhynchus rutili	P	0	0	0	0	0
Metabronema truttae	P	0	P	0	0	0
Cucullanus truttae	P	0	0	0	0	0
Crepidostomum metoecus	P	0	P	0	0	0
Phyllodistomum simile	P	0	0	0	0	0
Lecithaster gibbosus	0	0	0	4	0	0
Hemiurus communis	0	0	0	3	0	0
Brachyphallus crenatus	0	0	0	3	0	0
Derogenes varicus	0	0	0	37	29	22
Eubothrium crassum	0	0	0	50	50	60
Hepatoxylon sp.	0	0	0	12	9	4
Anisakidae	0	0	0	100	100	100
Salmincola salmonoides	0	0	0	85	79	81

P = present but exact incidence not determined.

The changes in the parasite fauna of migratory birds are even more complex. The fauna of swallows provides a good example, and has been studied intensively (Dogiel, 1964). Where the normal migratory pattern involves an extensive journey from the Northern to the Southern hemisphere, then four major groups of parasites can be distinguished:
1. Those that are ubiquitous. These are mainly ectoparasites, especially mallophagan lice. Some spend the whole of their lives on the bird, some are able to infect it in both hemispheres, and some survive the migration in the egg stage.
2. Southern parasites. These infect the birds only during their stay in the Southern hemisphere. They may complete their whole life cycle while the swallows remain there, or they may be carried to the North, where some die, or some may even complete the return journey.
3. Northern parasites. These are mainly those that infect nestlings or adults in the nest, and are chiefly fleas or other ectoparasites. Some die before the Southern migration, some are carried South and die there, and some return again. A small proportion remain in the nest in a quiescent state until the swallows return the following year.

4. Passage parasites. These are mainly digeneans, and are acquired en route during the migration.

In Russia, group 1 is the smallest, containing only 43 species, and group 3 the largest, with 300 species.

IN RELATION TO SEX OF HOST

Differences in parasite fauna between animals of different sexes are less common and less well understood. Most parasites are evenly distributed between the sexes, although for short periods they may show a preference for one. The infection of *Polystoma integerrimum* is higher in male frogs than in females just before the breeding season, as it appears that a high level of female hormones increases the host resistance to infection. The heavier incidence and abundance of the monogenean *Discocotyle sagittata* in male trout over the age of five was considered by contrast (Paling, 1965) to be the result of the greater attractiveness of mucus from males to larval oncomiracidia. The heavier levels of infection of *Mesocoelium monodi* in female lizards, however, were due to their larger appetites (Thomas, 1965) and to their eating more intermediate hosts than males. Clearly differences in distribution of parasites between hosts of different sexes are not due to any single cause but involve differences in host diet and physiology.

FREQUENCY DISTRIBUTIONS OF PARASITES WITHIN HOST POPULATIONS

Even within a single host age group or group with similar mode of life levels of parasite infection differ in different individuals. If the distribution of parasites within the host population were random, a frequency distribution of the pattern shown in Fig. 15A would be expected. This can be described by the Poisson model. Usually, however, the frequency distribution is far more similar to the pattern of Fig. 15B. This is typical of an overdispersed distribution, and whilst it can be described by several models, the negative binomial has generally been found to be the most satisfactory and to provide the best fit for helminth infections, and the Polya-Aeppli for protozoans. In fact, the distribution of the great majority of parasites in both their intermediate and their definitive hosts has been found to depart from random and to be capable of description by one of the models suitable for overdispersed distributions.

Such overdispersed distributions are likely to arise for a variety of reasons, all of which can be encountered in host-parasite systems. Heterogeneity in the probability of occurrence of the parasite is amongst the most frequent. For a random distribution every parasite must have the same probability of infecting a host, and each host must have the same probability of being infected. Any departure from this situation will lead to an aggregated distribution. In field situations it is very unlikely that this situation will obtain. Differences in the viability of larvae, and in the dispersion and behaviour of larval individuals will result in some parasites having a greater probability of infecting hosts than

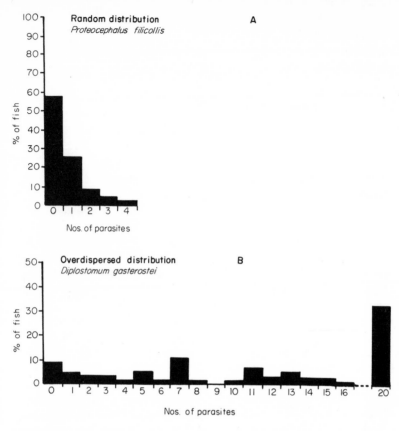

Fig. 15 Frequency distributions of parasites in their host populations: A. a random distribution (Poisson model). (Data from Hopkins, 1959); B. an aggregated distribution (negative binomial model). (After Pennycuick, 1971.)

others, and individual host differences in diet, susceptibility, behaviour and response to the parasite will ensure that some have a greater probability of being infected than others. Even when an apparently uniform batch of hosts are infected in the laboratory under standard conditions with the same number of parasites each, the variance in parasite numbers may exceed the mean (Table 29), a situation indicating overdispersion.

Overdispersion may also arise as a result of true contagion, where the presence of one individual in a host affects the probability of infection by another. This happens when the parasite is capable of asexual reproduction, since the presence of one individual leads inevitably to the presence of others, and when one individual so weakens a host that it is either more liable to infection by another or is less able to resist that infection. If infection occurs in random waves, but the mean number of parasites in each wave is high and the probability of infection changes from time to time, then overdispersion will again result.

Table 29 The mean (and variance) number of *Pomphorhynchus laevis* recovered from goldfish following different densities of infection. (From Kennedy, 1974.)

Mean no. of parasites administered	Weeks after infection					
	1	2	3	4	5	6
7	5.2	4.0	5.2	5.0	4.7	4.0
	(4.6)	(5.6)	(2.8)	(0.0)	(2.8)	(2.3)
14	13.0	10.0	11.5	11.0	11.6	9.6
	(20.0)	(8.5)	(7.1)	(18.3)	(17.1)	(1.3)
21	15.0	12.6	12.1	13.0	10.5	10.0
	(3.8)	(8.7)	(27.2)	(7.9)	(24.1)	(7.9)

In any host-parasite system therefore any differences in infectivity of parasites or susceptibility of host, whether having an ecological or physiological cause, will result in overdispersion of parasites throughout the host population. Since such differences are to be found in all natural populations it is not surprising that random distributions are so uncommon. The greater the degree of over-dispersion, the greater is the mean number of parasites for a given incidence of infection. This means that a large number of parasites occurs in a small number of hosts, and indeed most of the parasites may be concentrated into a very few host individuals. The importance of this with respect to the control of parasite numbers will be discussed later, but two implications deserve further attention. In the first place, overdispersion means that the flow of parasites through all the hosts in a population may not be similar. If the response of the host depends in kind or degree upon the intensity of infection, then different patterns of parasite flow may be observed and different controls operate simultaneously within the same host population. Secondly, and as a direct consequence of this, concentration upon a typical host-parasite system and the *mean* numbers of parasites per host may obscure important differences and be misleading. The *single* very heavily infected *individual* may be the important animal as far as survival and transmission of the parasite population to the next host is concerned (p. 86).

DISTRIBUTION OF INFECTED POPULATIONS

Since the factors controlling infection levels and the degree of overdispersion are likely to vary spatially, it follows that infected populations are likely to be distributed in a non-uniform manner in any locality. This situation has been studied in some detail by James (1968a and b, 1971), who examined the distribution of the digenean larvae in molluscs on rocky shores.

Adults of *Littorina saxatilis tenebrosa* are hosts to several parasites, and live in the upper littoral fringe of rocky shores. Twice a year, in early summer and winter, they migrate down to the lower supra-littoral fringe in order to give birth to their young. The adults and young, including those infected with the fluke *Parvatrema homoeotecnum,* then migrate back to the upper supra-littoral fringe. This ensures that although infection takes place only in the lower supra-

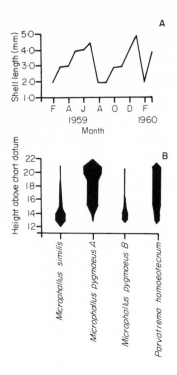

Fig. 16 Changes in the parasite fauna of *Littorina saxatilis tenebrosa*. A. changes in size group with highest percentage infection by *Parvatrema homoeotecnum*; B. variation in percentage infection by three species of larval digeneans with height on shore. (After James, 1968a.)

littoral fringe, parasitised specimens occur throughout the whole supra-littoral fringe, although the centre of infection moves up the shore (Fig. 16).

The other species of digeneans are, by contrast, restricted to well defined limits within the range of *L. saxatilis*. Specimens infected with species of *Microphallus* do not appear to migrate up the shore, due probably to the fact that young infestations grow rapidly and destroy the gonad of the host. Their distribution appears to relate to the behaviour of both the final and snail hosts. Thus, *M. pygmaeus A*, a parasite with no free-living stages, a single intermediate host and the herring gull as final host is common higher up the shore, where snails are exposed to infection for longer periods. *M. pygmaeus B* also has no free-living stage, only one intermediate host, and the rock pipit as a final host. It occurs only in juvenile host specimens, which are restricted almost entirely to the lower areas of the shore. The rock pipit is unable to feed on large snails and is also therefore particularly attracted to the lowest area of the shore, thus increasing the high incidence of the parasite there. *M. similis* by contrast, has a free-living cercaria, the crab as a second intermediate host and the herring gull as final host. The low tolerance of cercariae to exposure to air contributes to the restriction of this species to the lowest region of the shore.

The restriction of *P. homoeotecnum* to exposed shores may be due to the behaviour of its final host, the oyster catcher. This only occurs on shores with gently sloping supra-littoral fringes where the bird can perch whilst feeding. On very exposed rocky shores the snails are only found in very deep crevices or on precipitous rocks where the oyster catcher cannot get at them, and so does not visit the areas and distribute the infection there. The absence of the parasite from other sub-species of the host may be due in part to host insusceptibility but also because their shells are thicker and so are not normally eaten by birds, or if eaten pass straight through the gut. Thus James concluded that the distribution of infected populations could be due to the behaviour of the snail host, the behaviour of the definitive host, to host insusceptibility and to the effect of habitat conditions upon the free-living stages.

CHARACTERISATION OF HABITATS BY PARASITE FAUNAS

From what has been said previously it is clear that levels of infection may vary within a habitat. Nevertheless, several attempts have been made to characterise a habitat by its parasite fauna, and even to predict the occurrence of species and levels of infection. These attempts have been made particularly upon lake faunas, in an effort to characterise the parasite fauna of the different stages of lake succession. Wisniewski (1958) has studied a series of Polish lakes in great detail, and has concluded that whilst it is difficult, if not impossible, to predict the parasite fauna, it is nevertheless possible to recognise characteristic changes occurring in the course of lake succession. The greatest diversity of parasite fauna is found in oligotrophic lakes, where the majority of parasites complete their life cycles in fish. In such localities fish are the dominant predators, there are few terrestrial or avian predators serving as hosts to aquatic parasites, and the ecosystem is fairly closed. In eutrophic lakes by contrast parasite diversity is less, and many parasites complete their life cycles in birds. The parasites of fish are therefore often larval forms. There is considerable interaction between the lake and the surrounding area, and the system is much more open. These ideas have been confirmed by a similar study on the fauna of fish in Michigan by Esch (1971) (Table 30).

Table 30 Number of species from centrarchids in Michigan lakes according to the life cycle stage of the parasite. (From Esch, 1971.)

Stage	Gull lake oligotrophic	Wintergreen lake eutrophic	Duck lake eutrophic
Adult	10	4	2
Larvae of species completing life cycle in fish	4	0	0
Larvae of species completing life cycle in birds and mammals	3	4	4

Thus, in general terms, there is a characteristic pattern of parasite fauna in lakes of a particular status. In an aquatic ecosystem undergoing succession changes take place in the parasite fauna that relate to those taking place in the host fauna, and the parasites are going to be equally influenced by the factors influencing succession. Even in a mesotrophic lake it is possible to separate the oligotrophic and eutrophic elements of the parasite fauna (Chubb, 1963a). The parasite fauna is directly influenced by the feeding behaviour of its host and the trophic level of the latter, and the nature of the prey-predator relationships can therefore serve as a potential index for predicting the structure of the parasite fauna in any given aquatic ecosystem. It can not, however, be used to predict the details of the species present or their detailed host-parasite interactions.

ENERGY FLOW THROUGH HOST-PARASITE SYSTEMS

In an effort to understand the relationships between host and parasite populations, some recent attempts have been made to apply the principles and techniques of ecological energetics to host-parasite systems. The energy flow through any population can be expressed by the equations: energy of ingestion − energy of waste products = energy of assimilation, or

$$Q_c - Q_w = Q_g + Q_r$$

where Q_c =energy of food consumed per unit time, Q_w =energy of waste material (faeces etc.), Q_g =energy of growth and reproduction per unit time, and Q_r =energy of respiration per unit time. Since each of these terms can be measured for both parasitised and unparasitised hosts, the energy budgets of each can be determined and compared, and the overall effects of the parasite quantified. The attempts so far have been concerned with fish parasites.

An attempt to balance the energy budget of the *Schistocephalus solidus*—stickleback system was made by Walkey and Meakins (1970). Although respiratory expenditure by parasitised fish was greater than that of unparasitised, the variance recorded was very wide and the derived regressions of oxygen consumption upon weight of fish were not significantly different. Infection resulted in a greater depletion of host food reserves, shown by a marked increase of mortality of parasitised fish during starvation. When fed, differences in feeding and assimilation were found. Energy budgets were calculated for infected and uninfected fish over a period of one week. Despite the considerable variation observed, it appeared that the parasites exhibiting a high calorific incorporation rate caused a negative imbalance in the host energy budget, and assimilation rate was less than expenditure rate. In uninfected fish, fewer calories were expended in growth and respiration than were assimilated. Parasitised fish showed a higher gross efficiency, but the efficiency of the fish tissue alone, without the parasites, was lower than in uninfected fish, and the parasite was probably more efficient in its energy transformations than its host. Parasitised fish assimilating slowly ingested more food than uninfected fish. Host production was decreased by the presence of the parasite, and fish with a heavy load of small, rapidly growing parasites, could by depletion of host food reserves lose weight. The parasites therefore reduced fish production, the production: respiration ratio, and increased assimilation. This latter effect is undoubtedly due to the assimilation of the parasite itself, which, over a week, may exceed that of the host. Whether it would do so over the whole life span is not known, and possibly over a longer period host production may exceed that of the parasite.

The investigation of the *Caryophyllaeus laticeps*—annelid system was carried out in the field by Kennedy (1972), and did not attempt to solve the energy equation completely. Instead it attempted to quantify the effects of the parasite upon assimilation and determine the loss of production by the host population over the whole life span of host and parasite. Again, a wide variation in respiratory rates was noted, but oxygen uptake of infected and uninfected annelids did not differ significantly. Their growth rates, however, did (Fig. 17), and infected tissue grew at a slower rate than uninfected. Reproduction of annelids is also prevented by the presence of the parasite. Although it proved impossible to calculate absolute assimilation rates in the absence of information on respiration rates under natural conditions, relative assimilation rates and production values for infected and uninfected hosts could be compared (Table

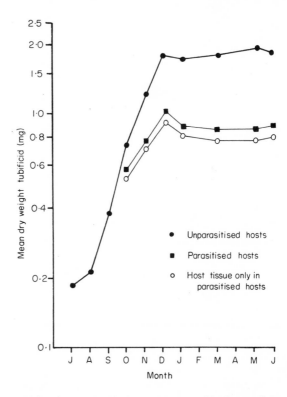

Fig. 17 Monthly changes in the mean weight of *Psammoryctides barbatus* parasitised by larvae of the cestode *Caryophyllaeus laticeps*. (After Kennedy, 1972.)

Table 31 Comparison of production and respiration of infected and uninfected *Psammoryctes barbatus* throughout life. (Data from Kennedy, 1972.)

Month	Uninfected tubificids				Infected tubificid tissue						C. laticeps	
	Production per time interval		Cumulative production	Respiration	Production per time interval		Cumulative production	Respiration	Loss of production		Production per time interval	Cumulative production
	(mg)	$(J = Q_g)$	(J)	$(J = Q_r)$	(mg)	$(J = Q_g)$	(J)	$(J = Q_r)$	(%)		(mg)	(mg)
July	+0.19	+4.47	4.47	k_1	+0.19	+4.47	4.47	k_1	0		0	0
Aug.	+0.02	+0.47	4.94	k_2	+0.02	+0.47	4.94	k_2	0		0	0
Sept.	+0.18	+4.24	9.18	k_3	+0.18	+4.24	9.18	k_3	0		0	0
Oct.	+0.34	+8.00	17.18	k_4	+0.14	+3.28	12.46	k_4	26.2		+0.0525	0.0525
Nov.	+0.48	+11.29	28.47	k_5	+0.19	+4.46	16.92	k_5	40.4		+0.0065	0.0590
Dec.	+0.59	+13.88	42.35	k_6	+0.22	+5.16	22.08	k_6	52.2		+0.0200	0.0790
Jan.	−0.06	−1.41	40.94	k_7	−0.12	−2.28	19.26	k_7	53.0		+0.0010	0.0800
Mar.	+0.04	+0.94	41.88	k_8	−0.05	−1.12	18.14	k_8	56.6		0	0.0800
May	+0.19	+4.28	46.16	k_9	−0.01	−0.22	17.92	k_9	61.2		+0.0100	0.0900
June	−0.12	−2.69	43.47	K	+0.02	+0.47	18.39	K	59.9		+0.0110	0.1010

31). The production of parasitised tissue is always less than that of unparasitised, and the loss of production due to the presence of the parasite is apparent as soon as the parasite is detectable. Over the life span of the host there is a loss of 60%, and even after six months it is as high as 52%. Since the respiration rates of infected and uninfected hosts can be represented by the same value, the production : respiration ratio of uninfected annelids is greater, by a factor of 2.5 times, than that of infected. Finally assimilation of parasitised animals must be less by a factor of 27.7 J, although the proportionate decrease in assimilation will be slight since energy expended on respiration accounts for a large proportion of assimilation energy.

In general, therefore, the effects of *C. laticeps* are both qualitatively and quantitatively similar to those of *S. solidus*. The major difference, the higher assimilation rate of parasitised fish, is due to the much greater rate of production of *S. solidus,* and as already noted, this may not be true over the whole life span of the system. It was also possible to calculate the effects of *C. laticeps* on its host population. Assuming a loss of production of 60% over the year for each infected host, then since only an average of 10% of the population is ever infected, the total loss to the population is only in the region of 6%. It is clear, therefore, that despite the pronounced effects a parasite may have on its individual host, accentuated by overdispersion, its effects on the host population may be very slight.

6 Parasite population changes in intermediate hosts

SYSTEMS IN WHICH THE PARASITE IS RELEASED FROM THE HOST

PARASITES IN VECTORS

In this type of system continual or irregular release of the parasite from the host is possible (p. 61 and Fig. 14A), and indeed is essential for the continuation of the life cycle. This will tend to reduce parasite numbers quite apart from any host response. It is also advantageous for the parasite not to kill the host. It might be expected in general terms therefore that the incidence of infection in a host population will continue to rise the longer that population is exposed to infection, whereas the mean intensity of infection will continue at a steady level as parasites are released or killed by host responses. The build up of infection levels will also depend upon the parasite's ability to reproduce asexually, which can counter the very low probabilities of infection experienced.

The most important factor governing the level of infection of protozoans in their arthropod vectors is the extent to which the vectors make contact with and feed upon infected mammals. This in turn is influenced by a large number of factors, including the availability and behaviour of the mammal, the feeding behaviour of the vector, and the climatic conditions (Gillies, 1972; Gatehouse, 1972). Most insect vectors have characteristic feeding and host location patterns of behaviour, which can be and are modified by climatic conditions such as wind and rain and by ecological conditions such as the presence and abundance of suitable mammals. In some cases the insects are able to travel long distances in order to seek out their prey, but in others they are restricted to very localised areas by the conditions there and their inability to fly far, and contact then depends upon the prey venturing within these areas.

Even when contact has been made with an infected vertebrate, infection is by no means inevitable. The parasite must be in the correct stage of its development to infect the vector, and present in suitable numbers. The successful infection of tsetse flies by *Trypanosoma gambiense* depends upon the parasite attaining a high level of infection in the mammal host and upon its being in the stumpy infective stage (p.117). Many parasites die in the intestine of the insect due to unfavourable conditions there, as they are especially sensitive to the acid : base ratio of the intestinal contents. Many others die in attempting to penetrate the peritrophic membrane of the vector, and this may well be responsible in part for the decline in incidence of infection with age found in many vectors. Tsetse flies, *Glossina palpalis,* were fed on a monkey infected with *T. gambiense* at various intervals after their emergence from pupation. The infection rate in newly emerged flies was

21%, in two day old flies 4% and in three day old ones 1%. In flies older than this infections could seldom, if ever, be achieved. It would thus appear that penetration is easiest just after the emergence of the fly when the peritrophic membrane is soft and discontinuous, and becomes progressively more difficult as the membrane hardens. Ookinetes of *Plasmodium gallinaceum* must also penetrate the intestinal lining of *Aedes aegypti* when it is soft, and this is only possible during the 30 hours after a meal, after which time the membrane hardens and becomes a barrier (Stohler, 1957).

The speed of coagulation of the blood in the intestine of the arthropod also affects the parasite: if this is slow the ookinete can penetrate any part of the wall, but if it is rapid the erythrocytes clot in the lower part of the mid-gut, leaving the serum and ookinetes in the upper part only. Development of the parasite is also affected by the temperature and by the nutritional state of the host. Variations in the diet of *Ae. aegypti* have a marked effect upon the number of developing *Plasmodium* oocysts, and low concentrations of bases or acids for example increase the susceptibility of the mosquito to infection whereas the salts of these bases increase resistance (Terzian *et al.*, 1956).

Within the host population there exists considerable variation with respect to susceptibility to infection. The differences in susceptibility of many mosquitoes to malarias are hereditary and have a genetic basis, and this is probably the most important single factor influencing the course of development of the parasites within the arthropods. The usual manifestations of it is that only a proportion of the mosquito population will harbour the parasite even when mosquitoes are exposed to heavily infected mammals. It has proved possible to breed susceptible and resistant strains of *Culex pipiens* to *Plasmodium cathemerium*. Huff (1929) found then when mosquitoes were allowed to feed freely upon infected birds only about 28% developed infections of the parasite, although zygotes and ookinete formation was observed in a much greater proportion. He then took eggs from the susceptible and resistant mosquitoes, bred them separately, and tested these adults for susceptibility. By repeating this process for several generations he was able to isolate a highly resistant strain with a 7.5% infection and a susceptible one with a 65% infection. The susceptibility appears to behave as a recessive Mendelian character, controlled by interacting multiple genes. Similar results have been obtained with other bird malarias (Table 32), but not

Table 32 Influence of selective breeding of mosquitoes on susceptibility to malaria infections. (From Garnham, 1964.)

Host	Parasite	Infective rates	
		Before selection	After selection
Culex pipiens	*P. cathemerium*	28%	65%
C. quinquefasciatus	,,	24%	59%
C. pipiens	*P. elongatum*	13%	49%
Anopheles quadrimaculatus	*P. gallinaceum*	20%	100%
Aedes aegypti	,,	100%	2%

as yet with mammal ones. A consequence of this susceptibility is that *Plasmodium* is very over-dispersed throughout the mosquito population, and this clearly has important consequences in relation to the probability of infection between vertebrates and vectors.

It appears that protozoans are relatively harmless to their vectors unless present in overwhelming numbers (Garnham, 1964). Death of the parasites is due chiefly to non-specific causes, and the arthropods are unable to acquire any immunity to subsequent infections. The cellular defence mechanisms of the hosts are employed principally against non-specific parasites (Tripp, 1969), and if employed against habitual ones are ineffective. The infections persist throughout the life of the host, and levels decline only when parasites are introduced into a vertebrate.

The relationship between filarial nematodes and their vectors appears to be fairly similar. Over-dispersion again appears to be due principally to differences in susceptibility of individual vectors to infection. These differences are also genetically based, and levels of infection seldom relate to the numbers of parasites acquired. Many larvae again die soon after ingestion and others fail to develop, so that there is very little mortality due to heavy infections amongst the vectors. In heavy infections larvae in all stages of development may be present, suggesting that infections have been superimposed upon each other and that there is no host resistance to re-infection. Larvae must also penetrate the intestinal wall before the membrane is secreted around the blood meal, and many fail to do so and are trapped. The number of larvae ingested is proportional to the level of infection of the vertebrate, i.e. to the number available and to the time of feeding, not to the volume of blood ingested (Table 33). If all the larvae ingested developed it would lead to heavy mortality amongst

Table 33 The level of infection of *Anopheles quadrimaculatus* with larvae of *Dirofilaria uniformis* when exposed to different levels of microfilariae in rabbits. (From Duxbury *et al.*, 1961.)

Microfilariae/ 0.02 ml blood	No. of mosquitoes fed	Mosquitoes surviving 10 days		Mean survival of mosquitoes in days	Mean no. of larvae
		No.	%		
95	39	25	64	6.6	23
253	37	18	49	5.4	21
310	53	23	43	5.8	22
3395	120	5	4	<1.0	74

the flies (Nelson, 1970), but in practice many fail to leave the mid-gut, and less than 50% of those ingested are generally able to escape from the intestine. This failure to escape from the intestine reduces most excess doses to supportable proportions, and the survival of most vectors is unaffected by the presence of the parasite. Super-infection is generally possible, but often the numbers establishing in the subsequent infections are lower (Table 34), and host responses are not effective against specific parasites.

Table 34 Effects of reinfection of *Anopheles quadrimaculatus* with *Dirofilaria uniformis* larvae upon infection levels. (From Duxbury *et al.*, 1961.)

| Type of blood meal | | No. of larvae recovered/5 mosquitoes | | |
Day 0	Day 10	1st infection	2nd infection	p
I (infected)	I	82	121	<0.001
N (not infected)	I	—	178	
I	N	50	—	
I	I	35	169	0.08
N	I	—	203	
I	N	98	—	

It would seem therefore that the level of infection of vectors by protozoans and nematodes is related principally to the levels of infection in the other hosts and to the probability of contact between vector and vertebrate, i.e. to ecological factors. These are often dependent upon climatic factors, especially high temperatures and humidity, and in temperate regions where climate changes seasonally transmission of the parasites may also be seasonal, and the levels of infection show seasonal changes. Following contact with the vector, the level of infection relates to the degree of heterogeneity shown by the arthropod population in susceptibility to infection. Death within infected hosts is not due to any specific response on the part of the host. This heavy, non-specific mortality serves to keep the infection levels low, although this may be compensated for amongst protozoans by asexual reproduction. If for some reason the probability of infection does increase drastically and parasite numbers rise to lethal levels, then the presence of insusceptible individuals within the host population ensures its survival. None of the factors reducing parasite numbers and infection levels appear to operate in a feedback manner, however, and so parasite-vector systems appear to be inherently unstable. This instability may lead to large local fluctuations in infection levels when conditions for transmission are favourable, and to the rapid rise, and fall, of infections to epidemic levels (Chapter 10).

DIGENEANS IN MOLLUSCAN HOSTS

In the course of infecting snails digenean larvae may experience considerable mortality, and only a small proportion of the miracida which make contact with and penetrate snails actually develop to the sporocyst stage. Penetration itself does little damage and provokes little response. It appears that in general snails respond to invaders in a non-specific fashion, and the miracidia that are able to infect are those that can block or overcome the response (Brooks, 1969). Preferred host species appear to be susceptible to infection throughout their life and no age resistance develops.

There is no simple relationship between the numbers of snails and the level of infection. Extensive asexual reproduction makes it in fact very difficult to estimate parasite numbers and the success of an infection. The rate of development and numbers of the parasite are certainly influenced by the food of the snail and by its size (Wright, 1971), since this generally indicates a good nutritional state. Well fed *Lymnea truncatula* produce between 133 and 344 rediae and 952–2275 cercariae per snail of *Fasciola hepatica* whereas after a comparable infection starved snails produce only 20–215 rediae and far less cercariae.

Competition may on occasion occur within the snail, since *Oncomelania quadrasi* produces no more cercariae of *Schistosoma japonicum* when infected with two or more miracidia than when infected with only one (Brooks, 1969). Infections in general persist throughout the life of the host and are seldom lost completely. Even during periods of host aestivation when many larvae die a few persist. Diminution of the infection level only occurs to any extent by loss of cercariae. This may be strictly seasonal, or release may continue over a long period. It has been shown that *Lymnea stagnalis* can lose its infection completely and recover from it, but this appears to be rare and most snails do not survive infection.

The developing parasites do affect their hosts (Wright, 1966b), and although acute castration is rare, reduced fecundity as a result of reduction in the size, number and viability of eggs is common. The growth of infected snails is frequently retarded, the shell is thinner and the glycogen reserves are depleted, which may affect the success of aestivation. In some cases parasitised molluscs may show accelerated growth and giganticism (Cheng, 1971), but the significance of this is not understood. The life span of infected snails is usually reduced, and they are less able to survive conditions of stress or extremes of climate. In most cases however the damage caused is moderate until cercarial emergence. Then the drain upon the snail's reserves, the fall in glycogen level and the mechanical damage inflicted during the emergence process may lead to premature death of the host.

There appears in general to be no barrier to re-infection of snails. Although it is difficult to demonstrate that re-infection has occurred, it is possible in the case of schistosomes. Infection by a single miracidium gives rise to adult flukes of one sex only. If individuals of both sexes are produced by a single snail then multiple infections must have occurred. It has thus been possible to show that re-infection following natural loss or loss during aestivation, and super-infection of *Biomphalaria glabrata* by *S. mansoni* can take place. Even a cellular response by the host to the parasite does not confer resistance to re-infection. When *B. boissyi* were exposed to miracidia of the Puerto Rican strain of *S. mansoni,* to which they are resistant, and then to the susceptible Egyptian strain no increase in resistance could be demonstrated (Wright, 1971). It appears also that some snails are able to secrete substances that immobilise miracidia (Wright, 1966a). Extracts of *B. glabrata* digestive glands and gonads prepared nine days after infection of the snail with *S. mansoni* had a marked immobilising effect upon miracidia of the same species. Between 76% and 100% of the treated miracidia were affected, whereas extracts from uninfected snails only immobilised about 22%, and extracts from other host species had no effect. The immobilisers were quite specific, and were not produced by snails carrying echinostome larvae. This would appear to be a mechanism for preventing super-infection, yet miracidia of the Caribbean strain of *S. mansoni* were immobilised by extracts of *Planorbis corneus,* an unsuitable host, and of the resistant Brasilian strain of *B. glabrata,* but not by extracts of the compatible and susceptible Caribbean strain of *B. glabrata.* It must be doubted therefore how far immobilisers are effective against the parasite strain from the same area as the host, and whether they do play much part in preventing super-infection.

The effects of the parasite population upon that of its host is much more difficult to determine, and depends upon the nature of the parasite and the time at which it infects the host. James (1965) compared the effects of five species of cercariae upon a population of *Littorina saxatilis.* The snail has a life span of 1C months and breeds twice in its life, at 6 months and 12 months old. The parasites affect both the digestive gland, by causing autolysis and depletion of reserves, and the gonads. Cercariae of *Parvatrema homoeotecnum* infect young snails only. They stop development of the gonad and hence breeding of the infected individual, and kill the snail after about 5 months. The other four species only infect spent adults after the young are born. *Cercaria ubiquita* infects most hosts after their second reproductive cycle. It destroys the gonad within a month and most of the digestive gland within two months, but infected snails live for about another four months. It thus has little or no effect upon the host population. *Cercaria littorina rudis* by contrast infects snails after their first reproductive cycle, and within four months the gonads are destroyed and the host killed. *Cercaria roscovita* infects after either breeding period, and kills the host within two months. *Cercaria lebouri* infects only after the first reproductive period and destroys the gonads, thus preventing second breeding. It does little damage to the digestive gland, however, and infected hosts live out a normal life span. Thus the effects of the parasites vary from the extreme of preventing infected snails from breeding at all to having no effect on reproduction of the host population. In each case the life span and time of cercarial release is appropriate to the length of time spent in the snail.

The level of infection in the host population may also vary seasonally, in a manner related to the breeding cycle, growth, migration and mortality of the host. James (1968a) has shown that the highest incidence of *Parvatrema homoeotecnum* in *L. saxatilis tenebrosa* is found in very young specimens, and that these also contain the youngest stages of the parasite. Reproduction of the snail in July and August is followed by a rapid rise in the incidence of the parasite, due to infection of the young snails. Infection levels increased from October to December, by which time the highest incidence occurred in rather larger specimens, due both to growth of infected individuals and to infection of snails that had hitherto escaped. From December to March the infection level fell rapidly, as a result of mortality amongst the now larger infected specimens. Reproduction of the snails in January and February was followed by a similar sequence of events in the parasite population, although the increase in incidence was less than that following the summer reproduction period. The centre of infection also moves up and down the shore in accordance with the movements of the snail population (p. 70).

The level of parasite infection in a snail population depends, therefore, to a very large extent upon the ecological factors influencing the probability of contact between host and parasite. In particular the nature of the habitat and the density of the snail population are of considerable importance. Infection levels tend always to be higher in ponds and well-defined water bodies, and to rise following an increase in the snail population. In some cases the abundance of the definitive host governs the level of infection (p. 134). In most localities the probability of infection is probably very low indeed (Hairston, 1965), and considerable mortality occurs amongst the miracidia. Further mortality takes place during the infection of the host. If infection is successful, the individual snail may carry large numbers of the parasite as a result of the latter's asexual reproduction, and this to some extent counters the heavy mortality of the infective stage. Clearly, as with vectors, specific host responses play little or no part in controlling parasite numbers, and again there appears to be no feedback control acting upon the parasites and so stabilising the host-parasite system.

Serious damage does not generally occur until cercariae are released, and although this may kill individual hosts, it will only affect their population if the level of infection is very high. This situation can always arise in an unstable system if conditions favour the parasite, but they rarely do so for long periods. If the parasite does seriously reduce the host population, then the probability of infection will decrease. This will permit the host population to build up again, followed by that of the parasite and so the cycle will be repeated. Over a long period of time therefore it might be expected that host and parasite populations will fluctuate in an irregular manner.

SYSTEMS IN WHICH THE PARASITE IS NOT RELEASED FROM THE HOST

In systems of this type transfer to the next host can only be achieved by ingestion of the intermediate host together with the parasites. Death of the host is thus essential, and provided that the parasite does not kill the host before the latter is ingested it is of no particular advantage to it to avoid damaging the host. The parasites may also be able to survive within the hosts for long periods, up to, in some cases, the life span of the latter.

CESTODES IN MAMMALS

Many mammals are able to employ immune responses against larval cestodes (Weinmann, 1970). Rodents infected with few or many cysts of *Hydatigera taeniaeformis* are virtually immune to oncospheres administered 56–105 days later. The immunity thus acquired develops very rapidly and persists for long periods. It is specific, and is associated with the early stages of invasion and curtails the establishment of new infections. The antigens provoking the response are probably produced by the hexacanth larva, since it is protective against the oncospheres but not the eggs. Even after removal of the cysts the immunity persists for up to 60 days. Transfer of serum from immune to non-immune hosts can confer immunity upon the latter which persists for 26 to 36 days, suggesting strongly that serum antibodies are involved in the protection. The response is only manifested in older hosts since the immune system is not fully developed or functional in young ones. The presence of the cysts may also induce local inflammation, but it is the immune response which prevents super-infection. Both sheep and cattle can also acquire strong and durable immunity to re-infection with cysts of *Taenia* species.

Not all mammals can acquire immunity to larval cestodes however. Sheep are never able to develop complete immunity to *Echinococcus granulosus* cysts, although fewer cysts establish and the host response is stronger in subsequent infections. There is also considerable variation in host response between individual sheep and between strains of sheep and parasites, and the successful development of cysts is influenced by the host response. In a few cases not only does the cestode fail to elicit any host response but its presence appears to be beneficial to the host. Thus, mice infected with *Spirometra mansonoides* gain weight up to 20% faster than uninfected mice (Mueller, 1968). The effect is additive up to 12 cestodes, and is due to a true difference in growth rate and not just to an increased food intake.

Since cestode cysts are usually capable of causing damage to their host tissues, the ability of mammals to acquire immunity prevents super-infection and its attendant dangers to the hosts. It is also an important cause of mortality amongst the parasites, and can clearly act as a feedback control upon parasite numbers. As these build up, only uninfected hosts can acquire new infections. Even if all the hosts become infected, the infection cannot exceed a certain level in each individual. Thus, whilst ecological factors may again determine the probability of infection and degree of contact between parasite and host, the level of infection is governed by the host response. This system is thus far more stable than those considered previously, and even if conditions favour the parasite, mortality of excess parasites due to the host responses ensures the persistence of both host and parasite populations with, probably, oscillations of a small and regular nature about an equilibrium position.

OTHER INTERMEDIATE HOST-PARASITE SYSTEMS

When the intermediate host is unable to respond to the parasite, incidence and intensity of infection tend to increase throughout the life of the host (Fig. 18A) as the time to which it is exposed to infection increases, resulting in more animals acquiring the infection and accumulating more parasites. Infection itself is often seasonal, since release of infective larvae is also often seasonal. This may cause a temporary rise in infection as recruitment exceeds mortality, but this then levels off again as recruitment ceases and heavily infected hosts are ingested.

Infections generally commence as soon as the ecological conditions permit contact between the host and parasite. Where the host has a short life span, infection is seasonal and the parasite does not kill the host, infection levels may rise initially and then level off. The annelid *Psammoryctides barbatus* has a life span of only a year. It is infected by the cestode *Caryophyllaeus laticeps* in June and July when the new generation of hosts first appears (Kennedy, 1969b), and both incidence and level of infection increase. Thereafter, however, further infection is impossible as the hosts age, infected and uninfected hosts are equally resistant to infection, and so both incidence and intensity of infection remain at the same level until death of the hosts occurs naturally after breeding in the following June (Table 35). Some intra-specific competition may take place amongst the parasites, and heavy infections of *C. laticeps* may be reduced in this way. Frequently, however, overinfection kills the host.

Table 35 Seasonal variation in the degree of infection of *Psammoryctes barbatus* by *Caryophyllaeus laticeps*. (From Kennedy, 1969.)

Month	D	J	F	M	A	M	J	J	A	S	O	N
% infection	11.4	10.6	8.3	8.3	8.4	14.7	27.2	7.4	6.8	8.6	9.9	6.4
MWB	1.1	1.0	1.1	1.1	1.0	1.0	1.0	1.1	1.1	1.0	1.0	1.0

Hosts may react to the presence of parasites by attempting to phagocytise or encapsulate them, and many parasites in their intermediate hosts are surrounded by a membrane or capsule of host origin. Whilst this seals off the parasite, it seldom destroys it. Since many parasites are in a resting state, the reduction of gases or nutrients due to the capsule has little or no effect upon them. In general only damaged parasites or parasites of the wrong species are destroyed by the host reactions.

Some parasites which do not kill their hosts are unusual in that their life span is shorter than that of the host. Perch serve as hosts for the plerocercoid larvae of the cestode *Triaenophorus nodulosus*. Infection is seasonal, occurring in May or June each year (Chubb, 1964). Incidence and mean parasite burden increase for the first two years of the host's life, but thereafter remain steady. The parasite is in fact only able to live in perch for 1.5–3 years, when it dies naturally and not as a result of any host response. Dead parasites are destroyed by the cellular activity of the host. The steady level of infection in older fish (Table 36) is thus the result of a state of equilibrium being achieved between seasonal recruitment and the degeneration of established parasites.

Table 36 Occurrence of plerocercoids of *Triaenophorus nodulosus* in the livers of perch. (From Chub, 1964.)

Month	N	D	J	F	M	A	M	J	J	A	S	O
% infected	70	53	42	56	71	65	72	70	40	35	38	30
No. of developing larvae/100 perch	0	0	0	0	4	11	17	4	0	0	0	0
No. of mature larvae/100 perch	70	100	100	100	96	94	76	90	72	95	92	100
No. of degenerate larvae/100 perch	30	0	0	0	4	3	37	26	33	5	8	0

In this type of system, and that of *C. laticeps,* therefore the level of parasitic infection depends almost entirely upon the number of parasites infecting the host. Competition and natural mortality may reduce the infection levels to some extent and even produce a state of equilibrium. Since the host's responses are unable to reduce heavy infections or prevent re-infection, there are no feedback controls operating, and the system is consequently unstable.

In a great many intermediate host-parasite systems the parasite has a deleterious effect upon the host, which is unable to respond effectively against it or prevent super-infection. The parasites are able to survive in the host throughout its life span, and again both incidence and intensity of infection increase with age. The effects of the parasite, however, become progressively more evident, and older and more heavily infected hosts tend to die off as a direct result of the infection. The mean parasite burden therefore declines amongst the older age groups (Fig. 18B). The parasites may also sterilise the hosts, and so contribute further to their population decline. The parasites may kill the host directly, or merely render them more susceptible to predation by the next host (p. 20).

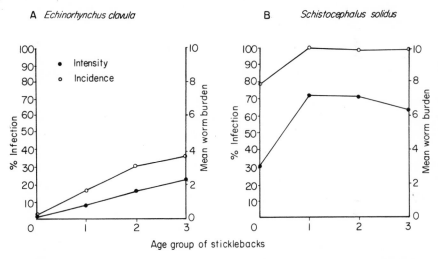

Fig. 18 Typical changes in the incidence and intensity of infection when A. the parasite does not affect its host's chances of survival; B. the parasite decreases its host's chances of survival. (After Pennycuick, 1971.)

The way in which this type of system is controlled and can be stabilised has been demonstrated by Pennycuick (1971) with reference to the parasites of sticklebacks. Both *Diplostomum gasterostei* and *Schistocephalus solidus* affected their host. Heavy infections of the digenean caused blindness, whereas the cestode affected growth, condition and breeding of the fish, rendered it more susceptible to predation and in heavy infections caused death directly. Both parasites were overdispersed throughout the host population (Table 37). Since *D. gasterostei* had less effect on the fish, its lethal population level was higher and its overdispersion greater, being described by a negative binomial model. The dispersion of *S.*

Table 37 Over-dispersion of parasites in sticklebacks. (From Pennycuick, 1971.)

	Diplostomum				Schistocephalus			
Date	% infected	mean	variance	$s^2/\bar{x}$	% infected	mean	variance	$s^2/\bar{x}$
IX.66	45.4	5.4	233.4	43.1	75.3	2.08	8.18	3.93
IV.67	18.9	0.7	8.2	11.5	84.9	5.66	98.3	17.35
VII.67	91.4	21.9	817.1	37.3	98.7	7.74	70.5	9.12
XII.67	66.1	20.5	1428.8	69.4	98.7	6.07	25.6	4.22

solidus was better described by a log series, which is more suitable for less heavy overdispersion.

Because of this overdispersion, a large number of parasites infected only a small number of hosts. Those most susceptible and most heavily infected died, and the effect of this was to reduce the parasite population by more individuals than the host population. Damage was therefore confined to a very few host individuals. The ingestion and death of a heavily infected fish thus has little effect upon the host population, but reduces the mean level of infection by the parasites considerably whilst at the same time ensuring successful completion of its life cycle.

The system is regulated in a manner that ensures maximum survival for the parasites and minimum deleterious effect upon the host population. For any particular set of conditions there is an optimum density of parasites per fish. Too many parasites per host may kill the host before it has a chance to be eaten, whilst too few hosts with large numbers of parasites reduce the chances of the next host locating them. Over a long term infection levels oscillate around this optimum density. If the parasite population is favoured by climatic or other conditions and starts to increase, mortality amongst the fish will also increase and breeding activity decline. Both will result in a decline in the host population, and, as the probability of infecting a host decreases correspondingly, in a decline in parasite numbers also. When these have fallen to a low level, the parasite's effects on the host population will be slight and the stickleback population can build up again, followed by that of the parasites. The complete cycle was estimated by Pennycuick to take 4–5 years in sticklebacks infected with *S. solidus*. The system is therefore essentially a stable one, with regular oscillations in numbers of hosts and parasites, since the controls operating upon it are doing so in a negative feedback manner.

STABILITY OF INTERMEDIATE HOST-PARASITE SYSTEMS

The most striking feature of intermediate host-parasite systems is the paucity of feedback controls operating upon the systems and their resulting instability. The incidence and level of infection of the parasite is determined in nearly all cases by the climatic or ecological factors influencing the probability of contact between host and parasite. With the conspicuous exception of mammals, which possess well-developed immune systems, mortality is seldom due to specific responses by the host against the parasite. Instead, low probabilities of infection, variation in susceptibility of hosts to infection and non-specific mortality during invasion prevent the build up of heavy infections. When these do occur, there is often no method of controlling them.

Overdispersion can minimise the effects of heavy infections by confining them to a few host individuals, and so the effect on the host population may be far less than would be predicted from the effects on individuals. The death of heavily infected hosts as a direct consequence of the presence of parasites may regulate parasite numbers and stabilise the host-parasite system by acting as a negative feedback control, but it is not at all clear whether this mechanism is actually widespread. It is undoubtedly effective where parasites habitually harm their hosts, but in many other systems the parasites seldom, if ever, probably reach a level where they are lethal since their numbers are kept well below this point by other mechanisms. Whilst therefore this mechanism may theoretically operate upon a great many host-parasite systems since most if not all parasites have a theoretical lethal level, under normal and natural conditions it is probably only effective with parasites that are fairly pathogenic. Only these therefore and mammalian cestodes amongst the whole range of parasites employing intermediate hosts or vectors are normally involved in forming systems stabilised by feedback controls. The remaining systems are fundamentally unstable, and even when they appear stable for long periods it is probably due to a fortuitous combination of climatic and ecological factors that themselves remain stable in the locality.

7 Population changes within poikilotherm definitive hosts

The parasites of poikilotherms have received far less attention than those of homoiotherms since few of them are pathogenic and fewer still are of any economic importance. There is consequently very little information available on protozoans, on the parasites of amphibians and reptiles, on parasites in tropical areas and on long-term parasite population changes. This chapter will therefore largely be concerned with the parasites of fish, and the short-term seasonal cycles in their parasite numbers.

MATURATION CYCLES

The majority of parasite species appear to be relatively short-lived in fish, and only *Diplozoon paradoxum* and one or two other monogeneans have been shown conclusively to live longer than one year in this host. The span of the remaining species varies from a month to about a year. Following a short period of establishment and differentiation immediately after infection, growth of the parasite commences but does not necessarily continue at a steady rate throughout the year. Whereas some species are able to grow and reproduce at any and all times of year, others are not. These are only capable of growth when certain conditions, climatic or otherwise, are favourable, and mature only when the parasite has attained adult size. Maturation in these species accordingly shows a seasonal cycle.

It is important to distinguish maturation cycles from seasonal incidence cycles, since there is no consistent correlation between them. Although all species which exhibit seasonal incidence and growth cycles also show seasonal maturation, species which are not seasonal in their incidence do not always breed throughout the year (Table 38). The same species may even exhibit different cycles in different localities. In Scotland *Proteocephalus filicollis* has a well-defined seasonal incidence cycle in sticklebacks, its growth is inhibited at cold winter temperatures, and it matures in late spring and early summer only (Hopkins, 1959). In Yorkshire, however, the same species in the same host does not show an incidence cycle and is able to grow and mature in all months (Chappell, 1969).

Where maturation is seasonal, the peak of egg production in temperate regions occurs almost inevitably in late spring or early summer, and the whole maturation cycle correlates closely with the annual cycle of water temperature changes. This general similarity in the time of maturation of different species in different hosts (Table 38) and the correlation with temperature suggests that the relationship may be a causal one (Chubb, 1967). This is not supported by any

Table 38 Maturation periods of some fish parasites.

Parasite	Host	Locality	Maturation period	Incidence
Echinorhynchus truttae	Trout	R. Terrig	All year	Non-seasonal
Acanthocephalus clavula	Stickleback	Bristol	All year	Seasonal
A. clavula	Grayling, Roach and other fish	L. Bala	All year	Non-seasonal
E. gadi	Cod	Barents Sea	All year	Non-seasonal
E. gadi	Cod	White Sea	Summer	Seasonal
Triaenophorus nodulosus	Pike	L. Bala	Late Winter–Spring	Non-seasonal
Neoechinorhynchus rutili	Stickleback	Durham	Spring	Non-seasonal
Proteocephalus filicollis	Stickleback	Glasgow	Spring	Seasonal
P. filicollis	Stickleback	Yorkshire	Spring peak	Non-seasonal

experimental evidence, however, and whilst it may be true for some species there must be considerable doubt in other cases. The differences in maturation of *P. filicollis* in different localities with similar temperature regimes strongly suggests that other factors are involved. The very precise timing of egg production in species such as *Mazocraes alosae* (p. 23) is also difficult to envisage as being controlled by temperature.

It has been demonstrated experimentally and unequivocably that maturation in the protozoans of amphibians, and *Opalina* and *Nyctotheres* in particular, have reproductive cycles synchronised with and physiologically controlled by their hosts (El Mofty and Smyth, 1969). During most of the year, when frogs are terrestrial, adult trophozoites are found in the intestine, and these reproduce occasionally asexually. As the breeding season of the host approaches and before the frog enters the water rapid division of the parasites takes place. Precystic forms produce cysts as the frogs begin copulation, and the percentage of cysts rises sharply following ovulation. Cyst formation is thus clearly associated with sexual reproduction of the frogs, and it can be inhibited by enforced hibernation of sexually mature frogs on land. Experimental injections of hormones into frogs confirms that the parasite maturation cycle is controlled by that of its host (Table 39).

Egg production in *Polystoma integerrimum* is also controlled by host maturation (p. 23), and egg production in many other fish parasites also correlates closely with host maturation. *Caryophyllaeus laticeps* matured in its host, dace, in the River Avon a month after the hosts, and when the hosts spawned a month later than usual one year the parasite also bred a month later (Kennedy, 1972). In other rivers the peak of maturation amongst the parasites occurred in April–May in dace, which breed in March, in May–June in chub, which breed in May, and in May–June in roach, which also breed in May. This correlation with host breeding and experimental verification that a rise in temperature alone is not sufficient to induce egg production in *C. laticeps* suggests that host hormones may also be involved, although maturation of the hosts themselves may be related to temperature cycles.

Table 39 Response of *Opalina ranarum* to injection of various hormones into its amphibian host. (From Smyth, 1962.)

	Normal	Pre-breeding season frogs Hypophysectomised	Gonadectomised
Pregnancy urine	+	+	−
Chorionic gonadotrophin	+	+	−
Serum gonadotrophin	+	+	−
Progesterone	−	−	0
Oesterone	+	+	−
Testosterone proprionate	+	+	+
Adrenaline	+	+	−

+ = cysts i.e. sexual reproduction present.
− = absent.
0 = not attempted.

Whatever their cause, seasonal maturation cycles can and do influence seasonality of incidence. The timing of maturation governs the timing of the appearance of the new generation of parasites, and if the one is seasonal, the other may also be, especially in species with a direct life cycle. In species employing an intermediate host, however, although production of the new generation may be seasonal, accumulation and persistence of later larval stages in an intermediate host may enable infective larvae to be available to fish all through the year and so eliminate or negate the effects of seasonal maturation. Since reproduction is also often followed by death of the parasite, seasonal maturation is frequently associated with seasonal mortality. This may then introduce seasonal trends into a cycle that does not otherwise show seasonal incidence. Thus maturation may influence the timing of both recruitment and mortality, and even though the factors causing maturation cycles may be independent of those causing incidence cycles, the two cycles may nevertheless be interdependent.

POPULATION CHANGES IN ECTOPARASITES

IN THE ABSENCE OF A HOST RESPONSE

Many fish protozoans do not appear to exhibit regular seasonal changes in incidence. Species such as *Trichodina* are present on fish of all ages and at all times of year, and they appear to be able to reproduce in all seasons. The major changes in their infection levels can be related to water temperatures and to the degree of aggregation of their hosts. All phases of development of fish protozoans, whether inducing a host response or not, are affected by temperature, and under warmer conditions generation time is much shorter (Table 40) and so the population size and infection levels are able to increase more rapidly. The success of transmission of the parasites is heavily influenced by the degree of crowding amongst the fish, and by the strength of the water

Table 40 The effect of temperature upon development time of *Ichthyophthirius multifiliis*. (From Bauer, 1962.)

Water temperature °C	26–27	24–25	20–22	17–18	15–16	11–12	7–8	4–5
Duration of reproduction (h)	10–12	14–15	18–20	23–26	28–30	36–40	72–84	144
Heat needed (° days)	13–14	15	16.5	17.2–18.5	18.6	18.6	24.5	25–30

currents (Bauer, 1962). When fish aggregate, as in spring for breeding and in winter shoals, infection levels rise, but when they disperse more widely for feeding, as tends to happen in summer, the level of infection declines despite the higher reproductive rate of the parasite. The effects of temperature and fish behaviour may thus cancel each other out, and lead to irregular changes in infection levels throughout the year.

Monogeneans, however, almost invariably undergo cyclic changes in incidence and abundance. Populations of *Dactylogyrus vastator* build up on carp in spring and summer and decline in winter (Dogiel, 1961). A few parasites remain on the fish over winter, and it is possible that some eggs also survive in the water. When the water temperature starts to rise in spring, these eggs hatch out and the overwintering adults produce eggs. Infection then commences, and as the temperature increases, each generation that infects takes a shorter time to reach maturity. There is thus a rapid and exponential rise in the parasite population size. The optimum temperature for breeding is around 20–25°C, and when the temperature falls below this level again in autumn, the rate of egg production and the generation time decreases and the population level falls again. At winter temperatures the parasites are unable to breed at all and so the population remains at a low level until the following spring. The related species *D. solidus* has a similar cycle but since its optimum temperature for egg production is only 15°C (Bauer, 1962) and eggs produced above this temperature are not viable, the timing of the cycle differs and the parasite reproduces and develops over winter.

In Crummock water *Discocotyle sagittata* has a similar cycle on char. The parasite lives for only one year, breeds and dies in summer, and the new generation infects fish in autumn (Paling, 1965). The same parasite in Lake Windermere, however, infects trout and appears to show no incidence cycle although the intensity of infection changes slightly in summer. In fact the parasite has a life span of between 3 and 4 years, and its persistence disguises the seasonal changes. Eggs are produced throughout the year, but they accumulate and remain dormant over winter at temperatures below 5°C. They hatch as the temperature rises in spring and give rise to a peak of infection in summer. Only a few of the parasites actually survive for 4 years and some die each year, especially in summer. Thus both recruitment and mortality are seasonal, but since both are restricted to summer and a proportion of the population persists on fish through this season, the incidence level only alters slightly and for a brief period.

IN THE PRESENCE OF A HOST RESPONSE

It is becoming apparent that in many cases of ectoparasitic infections fish are able to respond to the parasite, and may even acquire some degree of resistance to re-infection. This was first noticed in infections of fish with the monogenean *Benedenia melleni*. The parasite lives on the eyes of marine fish of the families Serranidae and Lutianidae. Under aquarium conditions heavy infections of the parasite built up to a level at which they killed some of the fish. If the fish survived, however, the level of infection declined. Despite being experimentally presented with opportunities, such fish were not subjected to re-infection (Nigrelli, 1935, 1937). It was also noted that infective larvae never settled at a site where a parasite had previously been attached. The mechanism of this acquired resistance is not understood, but it probably involves changes in the fish mucus which becomes toxic to the parasite and so renders the sites of previous infections unsuitable for later ones. *In vitro*, the parasites could survive for 3 days in saline, but lived 4–8 hours in mucus of unfavourable host species, 18–24 hours in mucus of susceptible but uninfected hosts, and a very much shorter period in mucus from susceptible infected hosts.

Host responses involving fish mucus are also known to limit infections by the protozoan *Ichthyophthirius multifiliis* (Bauer, 1962). The life cycle is very dependent upon temperature (Table 40), and numbers rise to a peak in summer and fall again over winter. The infection level is lower, however, when fish are re-infected although complete protection is never achieved (Table 41). The degree of

Table 41 Immunity of carp to reinfection with *Ichthyophthirius*. (From Bauer, 1962.)

Expt.	Control		Reinfection		Control/mean
	Mean intensity of infection	Range	Mean intensity of infection	Range	
1	105.4	41–305	10.4	9–24	14.5
2	180.2	114–370	16.6	2–43	10.8
3	7.8	1–25	0.4	0–1	19.5

resistance depends to a very large extent upon the density of the initial infection and varies considerably between individual fish. Resistance takes two weeks to develop but persists longer, and for at least two weeks after all the parasites have been lost. An individual fish can seldom be infected more than three times. As with the other ectoparasites, heavy infections may kill the fish, but carp exposed to a small number of parasites undergo a mild disease and recover during three weeks.

Infection levels of *Gyrodactylus* sp. on sticklebacks may also be controlled by host responses. Lester (1972) and Lester and Adams (1974) observed that the fish normally shed a layer of mucoid material from the skin every 1–2 days. When this is shed, the parasites are removed with it, apparently because the hooklets are attached to this slough instead of to the surface of the epidermis.

Slough was produced by uninfected fish, but increased in density in response to the presence of the parasite. The result of infecting fish with *Gyrodactylus* in the laboratory was an initial rise in level of infection due to reproduction of the parasite, followed by a sharp decline. Thus, after an initial infection of 20 flukes, the average number of parasites present at the end of successive weeks was 45, 68, 45 and 9. Fish re-infected within a week of their recovery lost all their

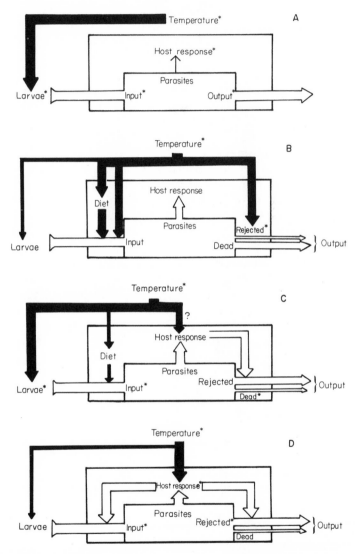

Fig. 19 Models of four types of poikilotherm definitive host-parasite system showing the parasite flow paths and probable control factors (solid lines). A. ectoparasites; B. non-seasonal endoparasites; C. seasonal endoparasites present all year; D. seasonal endoparasites present for less than a year. The thickness of the line indicates approximately the importance of the control, * that the factor varies regularly with time.

parasites within one week, if infected after two weeks harboured a small infection, and if fish were kept for four weeks before re-infection the parasites showed a normal cycle of rise and fall in infection level. The resistance to further infection thus lasted about three weeks. Where, for some reason, infection levels continued to rise after 2 weeks, death of the fish resulted. This happened naturally in some experiments but could also be induced by placing the fish under osmotic stress. The loss of parasites after two weeks was not due to any decline in their reproductive rate, but to an increasing number being shed with the slough. This shedding was unrelated to parasite age, but rate of loss was highest on the fish carrying the most parasites, and levels of over 100 parasites declined more rapidly than infections of 20–40. Thus individual fish showed fluctuations in parasite numbers and infection levels, controlled by a negative feedback host response. Nevertheless, because all the fish in any population are in different stages of resistance at any one time, the total population of parasites is probably more dependent upon temperature changes in a manner similar to other monogeneans, and host responses only regulate levels in individual fish and reduce parasite burdens to below lethal levels.

The great majority of ectoparasites therefore exhibit seasonal cycles in both incidence and intensity of infection, since maturation and generation time are so dependent upon temperature and upon seasonal temperature cycles. Although the populations increase in summer, the continual build up of heavy infections is prevented by changes in host behaviour or by a shortage of time when conditions for parasite population increase are favourable and the return of unfavourable conditions. Host responses may reduce the level of infection in individual fish, prevent the parasite attaining lethal densities, and alter the dispersion of the parasite throughout the host population. In this respect it can function as a negative feedback control upon population size, but it would seem that despite this, water temperature and host behaviour are the major controls upon the parasite population. These do not operate in a feedback manner, and so the system can be represented by Fig. 19A. It is fundamentally unstable, since despite the presence of host responses, long periods of favourable temperatures and host aggregation can and do lead to large increases in parasite numbers and epizootics involving death of hosts.

POPULATION CHANGES IN ENDOPARASITES

SPECIES NOT EXHIBITING SEASONAL INCIDENCE CYCLES

A number of fish parasites maintain a relatively constant level of both incidence and intensity of infection throughout the year. Although there may be irregular fluctuations in both parameters, there is no regular pattern of seasonal cyclical changes. Analysis of the changes in the composition of the parasites of *Triaenophorus nodulosus* in pike by Chubb (1963b) revealed that newly acquired parasites were present in fish in all months, and hence that recruitment was continuous throughout the year (Fig. 20). Although this tapeworm exhibited a

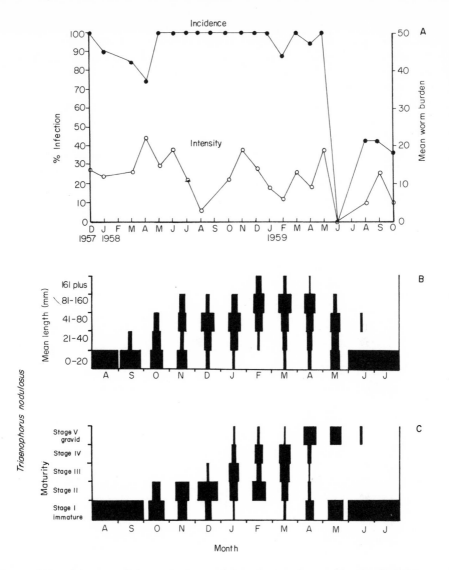

Fig. 20 The annual pattern of changes in the population of *Triaenophorus nodulosus* in pike in Llyn Tegid. (After Chubb, 1963b.)

well-defined maturation cycle, producing eggs only in late winter and spring, plerocercoid larvae could accumulate and survive in perch, the second intermediate host, for up to three years. They were thus available and infective to pike at all times of year. Since, however, recruitment was continuous yet the population size remained constant it must have been opposed by continuous and equal mortality. The cause of this was not known: the only mortality factor identified was the death of adult cestodes after breeding. The population was undoubtedly in a state of dynamic equilibrium between the gain and loss of parasites throughout the year, and the level of infestation and the fluctuations depended largely upon the extent to which pike fed upon perch.

The acanthocephalan *Pomphorhynchus laevis,* by contrast, breeds all the year round, as does its intermediate host *Gammarus pulex.* Acanthors are thus infective to *Gammarus* all year, develop within it all year, and so infective cystacanths are available to fish all year. Fish feed on *G. pulex* in all months, and so acquire the parasite throughout the year. The level of parasite infection in any individual fish appears to depend upon the extent to which it has fed upon *G. pulex.* If, therefore, the host's feeding habits are the most important influence upon recruitment rate, and hence population size, then since these alter throughout the year, seasonal peaks in abundance of the parasite might be expected. This does not in fact occur (Fig. 21), despite the fish feeding more intensively in

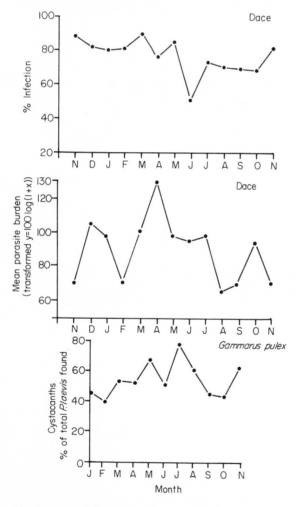

Fig. 21 Seasonal changes in infections of *Pomphorhynchus laevis* in the River Avon. (Data from Hine and Kennedy, 1974.)

96

summer than in winter. It has been shown experimentally, however (Kennedy, 1972), that although *P. laevis* is able to establish in fish at all temperatures, the proportion doing so declines as the temperature rises. Thus in summer when fish feed more intensively and acquire more cystacanths many of those ingested do not establish, whereas in winter, although the number ingested will be less as a result of the decline in feeding intensity and periods of starvation, more of those ingested are able to establish. Over the whole year therefore the influence of temperature upon host feeding intensity is opposed by its influence on the proportion of ingested parasites that establish, and the overall effect is to even out the seasonal variations in input by inducing a more or less steady rate of recruitment of parasites into the fish population.

In order to maintain the steady incidence observed throughout the year mortality must also be steady and equal, but temperature does not affect the survival rate after establishment and so cannot be responsible for equating recruitment rate with mortality rate. The rate of loss of parasites from the fish is not dependent upon the number ingested or established (Table 42), and although the fish may produce antibodies to the parasite, they are not effective against it. The

Table 42 The mean percentage recovery of *Pomphorhynchus laevis* following different densities of infection of goldfish. (From Kennedy, 1974.)

Mean no. of parasites administered	Weeks after infection					
	1	2	3	4	5	6
7	74.1	57.1	74.8	71.4	67.8	57.1
14	81.3	71.6	82.1	78.7	83.0	69.1
21	71.5	59.5	57.6	61.8	50.0	47.5
42	62.9	71.2	59.8	71.2	—	—

proportion of parasites establishing bore no relationship to the presence of an existing infection, nor could any evidence of intra-specific competition be found. The way in which mortality is equated with recruitment is therefore still unknown, as no feedback controls have yet been identified in this system. It seems probable that equation is a matter of chance, and the system inherently unstable. The apparent stability may in fact be due merely to a fortuitous combination of circumstances (Kennedy, 1974). Host diet and water temperature appear to be the major controls upon the flow of parasites through the system (Fig. 19B).

INDUCTION OF SEASONAL INCIDENCE CYCLES

In other systems, the effects of temperature and host diet may not act in opposition as they do with *P. laevis,* and seasonal changes in diet and availability of infective larvae and in parasite maturation can in fact result in seasonal changes in recruitment rate and so in levels of infection. The incidence of *Echinorhynchus truttae* in trout remains constant throughout the year (Awachie,

1965), but the level of infection shows seasonal changes and reaches a peak in July and August. Infective larvae are available all through the year, the intermediate host G. *pulex* is eaten throughout the year, and so infection of fish takes place all year. The occurrence of the infective cystacanth stage in G. *pulex* is, however, seasonal, and the intensities of parasitic infection in the intermediate and definitive hosts are inversely related. The low parasite levels in G. *pulex* in summer are here offset by the much higher feeding intensity of trout, and the parasite levels in fish actually rise at this time. In winter the heavier parasite burdens in G. *pulex* do not offset the greatly reduced feeding intensity of fish, and so the level of infection declines. Thus the level of the infection in trout depends upon the feeding intensity of fish and the availability of infective larvae, both of which change seasonally.

Seasonal changes are also evident in the infections with the cestode *Proteocephalus filicollis* in a Yorkshire pond (Chappell, 1969), although the incidence of the parasite remains fairly steady all year (Table 43). Although

Table 43 Seasonal variation in state of maturity of *Proteocephalus filicollis* in a Yorkshire pond. (From Chappell, 1969.)

	Month					
	Sept.	Nov.	Jan.	March	May/June	August
% gravid adults	48	32	39	31	33	46
% adults without eggs	30	19	11	28	44	36
% plerocercoids with early segmentation	—	6	3	10	14	9
% unsegmented plerocercoids	22	43	47	31	8	9
% incidence of parasite	34	49	48	48	45	55

infected copepods are available and are eaten all year, they are a more important source of food for the sticklebacks in winter, and new infections, exemplified by the incidence of unsegmented plerocercoids, are commoner at this time. The parasites grow and mature in all months, but there is a peak of maturation (gravid adults) in late summer. Since most parasites that establish survive to breed and then die, the greatest mortality factor, the loss of spent adults, is also seasonal. Host diet is again the major control of infection level, but its seasonal changes, indirectly influenced by temperature, and a seasonal maturation cycle amongst the parasites are inducing seasonal changes in the levels of infection.

SPECIES EXHIBITING SEASONAL INCIDENCE CYCLES

There is clearly no sharp distinction between seasonal and non-seasonal incidence cycles, and intermediate stages on the cline between them may occur when local conditions restrict infection periods or parasite maturation. It is rare, however, for a seasonal cycle to be due simply to seasonal production of eggs being followed by acquisition of new infections over a short period, as is often the case with ectoparasites. Seasonal inducing factors may operate to produce slight peaks in abundance in predominantly non-seasonal cycles, as discussed above, or to produce well-defined cycles in both incidence and intensity of infection.

In the River Ythan, *Podocotyle* sp. breeds all the year round in flounders, exhibits no seasonal cycle in incidence of infection, but shows pronounced seasonal changes in infection levels (Fig. 22). The cycle in fish is inversely correlated with the cycle in the second intermediate host, *Corophium volutator*, but directly with the cycle in the first intermediate host (Mackenzie and Gibson,

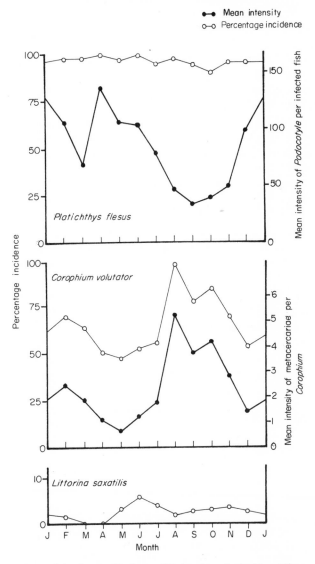

Fig. 22 Seasonal pattern of infestation of the three major hosts of *Podocotyle* sp. in the River Ythan. (After MacKenzie and Gibson, 1970.)

1970). The majority of eggs embryonate in spring, when the snail becomes infected. The parasites develop in the snail in early summer, cercariae are released in July and August, and *Corophium* acquires new infections in autumn. The increase in intensity of infection in fish after December is due not only to the availability of metacercariae then but also to the fact that *Corophium* is an important winter food of flounders, which feed upon it intensively at this time. In summer they feed upon a much wider variety of food, the older *Corophium* that harboured the infection in winter die off, the amphipod population is diluted by the appearance of young individuals that have not yet acquired the infection, and so the level of infection in *Corophium* declines. Thus changes in the availability of infective larvae, in the population structure of the intermediate host, and in the feeding habits of the fish result in a very restricted recruitment period and produce a clearly defined cycle in intensity of infection even when incidence remains steady.

Temperature may also play an important part in producing seasonal cycles. Cestodes of *Proteocephalus fluviatilis* only become gravid in small mouth bass between June and October, when water temperatures rise above 15°C. Eggs infect copepods in summer, and plerocercoids begin to appear in fish in late summer. Once in the fish they begin to develop, and if they infect early in a warm summer may become gravid by September (Fischer, 1967). More often they do not produce eggs by winter, and their development is then halted until temperatures rise in spring. Eggs produced in winter and late autumn are killed by the low winter temperatures, infection of neither host is then possible, and so infection levels in fish fall.

Temperature may influence population changes in still other ways. Plerocercoids of *Proteocephalus ambloplitis* are found in the viscera of small mouth bass at all times of year, but incidence of infection in the intestine is seasonal (Fischer and Freeman, 1969). The infection level in the intestine rises to a peak in spring then declines in summer when the cestodes die after breeding, and falls to zero over winter. When bass containing visceral plerocercoids were taken from a lake at 4°C in winter and maintained in the laboratory at 7°C and over, the plerocercoids migrated from the viscera to the intestinal lumen (Table 44). This occurs naturally in the lake in May and June to produce the spring rise in incidence. If

Table 44 Effect of raising temperature of the small-mouth bass kept over winter at 4°C. (From Fischer and Freeman, 1969.)

Temp °C	No. of plerocercoids penetrating	in gut	No. of segmented worms in gut
5.5	0	0	0
5.5	0	0	0
7	10	34	0
7	3	9	0
10	2	42	0
10	1	33	1

bass eat forage fish containing plerocercoids in summer, the larvae do not remain in the intestine but are either lost or move into the viscera. Temperature thus prevents the establishment of intestinal infections in summer and winter, and by restricting recruitment causes a seasonal incidence cycle.

The incidence of *Proteocephalus filicollis* in sticklebacks in Scotland, as opposed to Yorkshire (p. 98) is also seasonal (Hopkins, 1959). Infection commences in June, reaches its maximum level between August and December and then declines (Fig. 23). This is not, however, a simple cycle of summer infection,

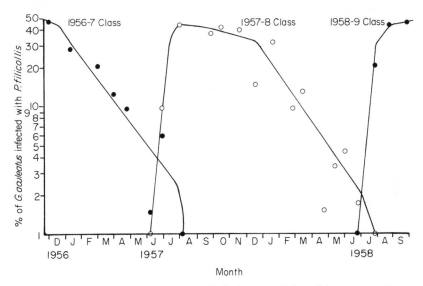

Fig. 23 Seasonal incidence cycle of *Proteocephalus filicollis* in a population of *Gasterosteus aculeatus*. (After Hopkins, 1959.)

winter growth and spring death. Loss of parasites from the fish commences immediately after infection, and continues at a constant rate throughout the year. In fact less than 1% of all the parasites infecting fish survive to produce eggs. Apart from the loss of spent adults, mortality is not seasonal. Between July and November infective larvae are available and the rate of infection by parasites exceeds the rate of loss. After November, when recruitment stops, the constant rate of loss is evident, and the infection level declines. The changes in infection levels are therefore cyclical because recruitment period is restricted. This in turn depends upon the maturation cycle, which is temperature controlled, and the availability of intermediate hosts, which is also affected by temperature. The system can be represented by Fig. 19C.

The cestode *Caryophyllaeus laticeps* shows a very well defined cycle in both incidence and intensity of infection of fish of the River Avon. Infection commences in December, incidence reaches a peak in February, and the level declines and parasites disappear from the fish in July (Kennedy, 1969b). Changes in incidence and population structure (Fig. 24) showed that infection took place between December and March, and that mortality commenced certainly as early as March and probably earlier. Thus in the colder months infection rates exceeded mortality, but in spring when infection ceased, mortality continued and the parasites soon disappeared. Mortality changes were not seasonal, and so not responsible for the observed cycle. The restricted recruitment

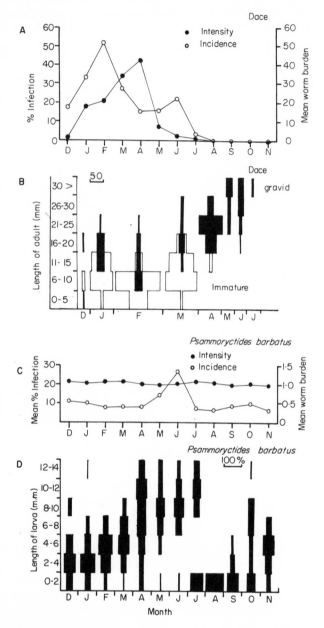

Fig. 24 The annual pattern of changes in the population of *Caryophyllaeus laticeps* in the River Avon. (After Kennedy, 1969.)

period of *C. laticeps* was not due to seasonal availability of infective larvae, which were present at a relatively constant density for the greater part of the year. Experimental studies have shown that *C. laticeps* can establish in fish more readily and survive for longer periods at low temperatures (Kennedy, 1971). At warm temperatures the fish reject the parasites after a few days. It was thus suggested that infection was only possible in the river at the low winter temperatures, and as the water temperature rose new infections were no longer possible and existing infections were eliminated. Temperature, therefore, bore a causal relationship to the infection cycle, and was clearly the major control factor (Fig. 19D). In other localities, where the temperature regime is different, fish may not feed in winter and so the timing of the cycle also differs.

In none of the endoparasite systems considered so far has there been any evidence that host responses directed specifically against the parasites are important controls upon the system. This has, however, been suggested as an explanation for the population changes of *Gyrocotyle* sp. in *Chimaera* (Halvorsen and Williams, 1968). The incidence of infection by the parasite is age dependent, but whereas young fish may carry large numbers of parasites, most older fish carry only a single pair (Table 45). It is suggested that these two form a sexual

Table 45 Number of *Chimaera* from different length groups infected with *Gyrocotyle*. (From Halvorsen and Williams, 1968.)

No. of *Gyrocotyle*	Length of *Chimaera* (cm)						
	13–20	20–25	25–30	30–35	35–40	40–45	60–85
0	16	0	2	1	0	0	0
1	1	10	8	3	0	0	1
2	0	4	7	5	4	4	8
3	0	0	1	0	0	0	1
4	0	2	0	0	0	0	1
>4	1	2	1	0	0	0	0

unit, and that whereas young fish take in an initial infection of many larvae, only two survive and succeed in establishing and growing to maturity. Premunition and crowding were excluded as explanations of this situation, and intrinsic regulatory factors of unknown identity, based on host responses, were postulated as causes.

REGULATION AND STABILITY OF POIKILOTHERM DEFINITIVE HOST-PARASITE SYSTEMS

It is clear from what has been said that the levels of infections of parasites in poikilotherm definitive hosts is determined largely by the factors that influence the rate of infection of the fish. These may involve either the behaviour of the fish or its diet, but both in turn are affected directly by habitat temperature.

Annual changes in water temperature may determine that the rates of infection change in a regular seasonal manner by controlling the reproductive period of the parasite, the availability of infective larvae, the establishment of the parasite, host food preferences or host behaviour and so induce regular seasonal cycles in infection levels. By contrast changes in parasite mortality rate appear to have very little effect upon the pattern of changes in infection levels. Seasonal mortality may reinforce cycles governed primarily by other factors. Specific host responses may in some cases reduce infection levels in individual fish, but mortality rates, with one or two possible exceptions, appear to be independent of infection rates or infection levels. There is very little evidence that mortality acts as an important feedback control under most natural conditions.

Indeed, in the majority of poikilotherm definitive host-parasite systems studied to date there is no indication at all of the existence of feedback controls that could stabilise the system and control infection levels. Where infection levels remain stable over long periods, this appears to be due to the stability of the ecological conditions in the habitat. Where they change in a regular manner, this is due to the regularity in the changes of climatic factors and habitat conditions. In the present state of knowledge, therefore, these host-parasite systems appear in many cases to be unstable. It is not surprising, then, that the pattern of changes in a system is not characteristic of that particular system or of a particular time, but changes from place to place and time to time as local conditions alter.

8 Population changes within bird definitive hosts

IMMUNE RESPONSES OF HOMOIOTHERMS

Homoiotherm host-parasite systems differ principally from those of poikilotherms in that host responses to the parasite play a far more important part in effecting parasite mortality. The immune systems of homoiotherms are better developed, function over a wider range of conditions and are more effective, and a great many parasites of homoiotherms invoke immunological responses directed specifically against them.

The effects of the immune responses upon the parasites varies, not only from system to system, but also within any system in relation to the age of the host, its condition and the strain of the parasite. The immune system is generally not fully functional in young animals, these are more readily infected, and then age resistance, due to host defence mechanisms, appears. The general condition and diet of an animal also influences the effectiveness of its immune responses, and different strains of parasites may possess different antigens.

An immune response may result in elimination of the parasite that provoked it and/or may make the host refractory to re-infection. Other manifestations include a reduced rate of establishment on subsequent infection, stunting of parasite growth, reduced fecundity or inhibition of reproduction, and retardation of development and increase in generation time (Sprent, 1969). If, as Dineen (1963) suggests, there is also a threshold level of antigen needed to stimulate a response and this depends upon the degree of antigenic disparity between host and parasite and the level of information flow, then the nature and strength of the response will vary between hosts, and in any host will depend on the infection level and may only be manifested at all above a threshold level of parasite density. Even then, many parasites are capable of avoiding the immune responses they provoke. Immune responses are, however, capable of operating in a negative feedback manner, and of controlling infection levels and population size rather than just eliminating the parasites. This is clearly of advantage to the parasite and to the host-parasite system. The exact mechanism of the response and especially the relative importance of circulating antibodies and hypersensitivity reactions is frequently obscure. In the present context, however, it is the effectiveness rather than the mechanism that is important, and it is necessary to concentrate upon the functional aspects and the manifestations of the hosts' responses.

The parasites of homoiotherms have, in general, received far more attention than those of poikilotherms. Because of their medical and veterinary importance, however, much of the information available relates only to relatively few hosts, primarily to man and his domestic animals. Many of the

105

studies of domestic animals in particular have been carried out under farm or experimental conditions, and relatively little is known about parasite population changes in wild animals under natural conditions. This chapter and the next will therefore be concerned with a limited range of host and parasite systems only, many of which exist under atypical or unnatural conditions.

PROTOZOAN PARASITES OF DOMESTIC BIRDS

So far as is known most birds develop some degree of resistance to re-infection with protozoan parasites. Amongst the most studied of the bird protozoans is *Eimeria,* the causative agent of avian coccidiosis. Infections of *Eimeria* spp. are self terminating since the parasites cannot multiply indefinitely and the oocysts must be shed from the host for the life cycle to be completed. Following infections of chickens with *E. acervulina,* the production of oocysts rises until the fifth or sixth day and then declines (Table 46), the exact time depending upon the size of the initial infection (Joyner, 1969). The heavier the initial infection, the later the date of maximum oocyst production and disappearance of the infection.

Table 46 The average daily output in millions per bird following the infection of 13-day-old chicks with different numbers of oocysts of *Eimeria acervulina.* (From Joyner, 1969.)

	Oocyst dose (thousands)			
Day	1.25	20	320	5120
4	+	+	0	0
5	8	140	37	2
6	43	68	79	1
7	9	28	46	+
8	2	18	37	1
9	1	5	14	4
10	1	3	6	25
11	+	+	1	32
12	0	+	+	20
13	0	+	+	3
14	0	0	+	+
Total	64	262	220	88
Oocysts produced/ oocyst inoculated:	51,200	13,100	687	17

+ = barely detectable.
0 = undetectable.

The numbers of oocysts produced in any *Eimeria* infection are dependent upon a number of factors. These include the reproductive potential of the parasite, which varies from species to species (Table 2), and from strain to strain within a species. Strain M of *E. acervulina,* for example, consistently produces more oocysts than strain W (Table 47). These differences of reproductive

Table 47 The average daily output in millions per bird following the infection of chicks with different numbers of the two strains of *Eimeria acervulina*. (From Joyner, 1969.)

		Oocyst dose (thousands)				
		80	320	1280	5120	20480
Total production	Strain W	283	220	88	88	62
after 14 days of	Strain M	918	650	480	252	215

potential between species or strains lead to differences in the manifestation of the infections. *E. tenella,* which has a high reproductive potential and is pathogenic, kills young chickens, whereas *E. necatrix,* which is equally virulent but has a lower reproductive potential, causes disease in older birds. *E. acervulina,* with a high reproductive potential but with low virulence, has to be present in enormous numbers to cause disease. The degree of crowding is also important in influencing oocyst production, and there is clearly an optimum level of infection which produces the maximum number of oocysts per initial infection (Tables 21 and 22, pp. 53–54). Oocyst production may also be affected by the level of immunity developed by the host, the nutritional state of the host, its age and strain, and the presence of other species of *Eimeria* (p. 58) (Williams, 1973).

Following an initial infection with a species of *Eimeria,* birds become partially or completely immune to re-infection. The degree of immunity shown depends upon the age of the bird and the size of the initial infection, complete immunity only appearing after very heavy infections. Chickens infected with *E. acervulina* were re-infected with doses of oocysts of increasing size at two-weekly intervals, and within 14 days the birds had developed almost complete immunity to re-infection (Table 48). A single exposure to the parasites may therefore be enough to induce complete resistance to re-infection. In other species only partial resistance develops after a single infection, and exposure to two or three infections is necessary to stimulate complete immunity.

Chickens may remain immune for from 2 to 6 months, depending upon the size of the initial infection and species, and they can acquire specific immunity to each species of *Eimeria* (p. 58). In an immune host the sporozoites are affected

Table 48 The immunisation of chicken to a homologous strain of *Eimeria acervulina*. (From Joyner, 1969.)

		Group 1		Group 2	
Day	Infection no. of oocysts	Total oocyst production per bird	Patent period (days)	Total oocyst production per bird	Patent period (days)
0	80,000	295×10^6	10	338×10^6	10
14	160,000	few	1	few	3
28	5.12×10^6	few	1	few	2

after penetrating the epithelium. They may encyst but do not develop in immune cells. Partial immunity is manifested by the production of a reduced number of oocysts. The immune response occurs in the intestine (Cuckler, 1970), at the cellular level, although in conjunction with protective humoral antibodies. Thus, if a bird recovers from an initial infection of *Eimeria*, the partial or complete immunity developed by the host keeps the parasite infection level in any subsequent infection at a very low density.

The response of chickens to continuous low levels of infections with *Eimeria*, a situation which approximates more closely to natural as opposed to domestic situations, has also been investigated (Joyner and Norton, 1973). Chickens receiving daily doses of 5 oocysts produced almost the same total number of oocysts as birds receiving a single dose of 100, although the patent period of infection was twice as long in the former case (Table 49). Uninfected chickens

Table 49 Oocyst production in chickens infected with 5 oocysts of *Eimeria tenella* daily or with a single dose of 100 oocysts. (From Joyner and Norton, 1973.)

Regime	Total oocyst production over 28 days	Duration of patency (days)
5 per day	7.47	20
100	7.67	10

and chickens given a single infection of 5 oocysts were killed by an infection of 50,000 oocysts. Birds given a single dose of 100 oocysts were only partially immune to re-infection, and 6 out of 10 died, whereas the birds given a daily dose of 5 oocysts per day for 28 days survived. Thus, not only may repeated low level infections confer immunity upon chickens, but the immunity may be more effective than that produced in birds receiving a single dose. Thus, under natural conditions, it might be expected that most birds over 6–10 weeks of age will be immune to infection and will carry very low parasite burdens. It is clear therefore that infection levels of *Eimeria* in individual birds can be regulated in a negative feedback manner by both host immune responses and by intra-specific competition. The size of the whole parasite population can thus be controlled by the host.

Immunity is also exhibited by birds to avian malaria, although this appears to be of the premunition type where the continued presence of the parasite is necessary to stimulate the immune response (McGhee, 1970). Although haemolysis is associated with a decline in *P. lophurae* infections in ducks, humoral antibodies are very hard to demonstrate in *Plasmodium* infections and are probably not very effective. The lymphoid/macrophage system is, however, undoubtedly involved. Under experimental conditions several repeated doses are better for stimulating immunity than a single massive one, but it appears that under natural conditions acquired immunity may be of little importance in regulating infection levels or the parasite population. Both incidence, and to some extent intensity, of infection appear to be determined instead by ecological factors that determine the degree of contact between the arthropod vector and the bird host.

NEMATODE INFECTIONS OF DOMESTIC BIRDS

The establishment of nematode infections in chickens is dependent upon the age of the bird and the size of the infection dose. Ackert (1942) was able to demonstrate that chickens became increasingly resistant to infections with *Ascaridea lineata* with age, and that this appeared to be due to a substance present in the intestinal mucus which inhibited nutrition of the larvae and became more effective in older chickens as the number of mucus cells increased rather than to any specific response by the birds to the parasite. The proportion of any infective dose establishing is also related to the size of the dose (Table 50), being higher at lower levels of infection, although there was considerable variation in the rate of establishment between individual birds. The size of individual nematodes was also greater in the lower infections.

Table 50 The survival of *Ascaridea lineata* in chickens following different levels of infection. (From Ackert *et al.*, 1931.)

Infection dose	500	300	100	50	25
Mean nos. surviving	13.21	11.63	9.66	5.97	5.73
% surviving	2.6	3.9	9.6	11.9	22.9

Nematode infections may also provoke resistance in their bird hosts. Chickens of 5 weeks old were infected with *Heterakis* sp. and given a second infection 28 days later (Lund, 1967). The initial immunising dose was unaffected by the challenge, but the second infection suffered a 37% reduction in establishment compared with the controls. In turkeys of the same age and infected on the same occasions both the immunising and second (challenge) doses were reduced by 40% following challenge. When eggs of *Ascaridia galli* were administered to chickens at a rate of 10 and 1000 eggs per day respectively, larvae arrested in development accumulated in birds receiving the higher dose (Table 51). Sporadic development of these to the adult stage occurred later (Ikeme, 1971). This development inhibition does not appear to be related to the size of the parasite population, since it also occurred in single infections of 1000 eggs, and is probably a manifestation of host resistance. Infections of 10 eggs per day provoked no response by the host and no more control than a single primary infection, but as the infection rate increased up to 1000 a day, not only did retardation occur, but also egg output was delayed, depressed or suppressed. There is not therefore a cumulative build up of parasites nor a regular turnover in infections since development and reproduction are inhibited at high densities, generation time is prolonged, and so the parasite numbers are regulated to some extent by the host response. This again functions in a feedback manner, but appears to be less effective than responses to bird protozoans.

Table 51 Infection levels of chicken with *Ascaridia galli* following infections of 10 and 1000 eggs per day. (From Ikeme, 1971.)

Week	10 eggs per day					1000 eggs per day				
	2nd stage larva	3rd stage larva	4th stage larva	Total larvae	adult	2nd stage larva	3rd stage larva	4th stage larva	Total larvae	adult
1	233	33	—	267	0	900	0	0	900	0
2	199	166	—	396	0	5667	2534	0	8200	0
3	99	300	66	365	10	3666	2434	0	6,100	0
4	66	200	66	332	10	1800	2193	0	4000	0
5	66	266	99	431	28	33	2266	0	2299	0
6	66	133	99	298	42	0	2133	0	2133	0
7	66	100	66	232	62	0	2133	0	2166	0
8	0	0	0	0	62	0	2533	0	2533	0

TAPEWORMS OF DOMESTIC BIRDS

The course of the infection of the cestode *Raillietina cesticillus* has been studied experimentally in chickens in some detail (Gray, 1972a, b, 1973). Following infection, the cestodes migrate down the alimentary tract, and a proportion of them are lost in the process. The remainder attach in their preferred site, and commence proglottid production at 12 days. With infections of 100 cysticercoids per bird a rapid rise in the rate of proglottid production occurs initially which then levels out at about 20 days to an output of between 120 and 200 proglottids per bird per day. After 39 days a slow decline in the rate of output sets in. At 56 days the number of scolices, i.e. tapeworms, starts to fall, until at 112 days very few parasites remained. Closer study of the parasites themselves showed that at 28 days a small proportion of parasites had lost all or part of their strobilae, and this process continued until at 70 days almost all the cestodes had destrobilated and thus the infection was effectively self-terminating at 70 days, despite the persistence of scolices. These did not regenerate strobilae, and were eventually lost. When infections of different sizes were administered, crowding effects were evident. Destrobilation could also be induced by starving the birds, though regeneration of strobilae was then possible when birds were returned to a normal diet. Chickens also became more resistant to the cestode with increasing age, manifested by a decreased rate of establishment and growth, an increased rate of destrobilation and a consequent loss of scolices.

When infected birds were exposed to re-infection following elimination of the initial infection, the tapeworms were able to establish in the chickens at the same rate, but they failed to grow mature strobilae (Table 52). The chickens were thus clearly able to acquire a resistance to the infection which, moreover, persisted even in the absence of the primary infection. This resistance could be inhibited by the use of immunosuppressant drugs. If scolices from resistant birds were transplanted to uninfected chickens they were able to regrow their

Table 52 Resistance of chickens to infection with *Raillietina cesticillus*. (From Gray, 1973.)

Group of hosts	Mean no. of scolices	p	Mean % no. of scolices without strobilae	p
Reinfected male	16.9		94.63	
		>0.05		< 0.001
Control male	20.9		67.31	
Reinfected female	9.8		100.0	
		>0.001		< 0.001
Control female	24.3		56.56	

strobilae, thus indicating that the loss of strobilae in an immune environment is a reversible process. The inflammatory response found around the scolices in secondary infections was also inhibited by the drug.

Thus, *R. cesticillus* clearly provokes an immune response by its hosts, and this contributes to the loss of strobilae by parasites. Non-specific factors involving deterioration of the intestine as an environment are also involved, however, which the immune responses simply amplify. Nevertheless, it is evident that host resistance factors as well as crowding operate to affect the parasites, and the effect is manifested by reduced proglottid formation and hence reproductive rate rather than by an immediate reduction in numbers, although this follows later. The parasite numbers can therefore be regulated in a feedback manner directly related to the size of the infection.

CESTODES OF WILD BIRDS

The changes in structure and size of the cestode infections were studied by Avery (1969) in ducks exposed under natural conditions to repeated invasions by cysticercoids of *Sobolevicanthus gracilis*. At first the infection comprised a small number of large, mature cestodes, then the mean level of infection rose and this changed to a large number of small, stunted and immature cestodes, and eventually the number of parasites declined. For the first 18 to 56 days the size of the parasites was inversely proportional to the number present, indicating the occurrence of intra-specific competition. After the 56th day, all parasites were small and their size was no longer related to the density of infection (Fig. 25). Growth, and hence maturation and egg production, was evidently inhibited after continuous exposure of ducks to high levels of infection. This was not due to overcrowding nor to food shortage amongst the ducks. The inhibition occurred earlier at higher densities, and appeared to be due to a change in the suitability of the host provoked by the initial infections, which were themselves able to grow and mature normally. Whatever the mechanism, it appears to reduce the effects of high densities of parasites and limits the rapid increase in the cestode population which would occur when ducks aggregate by reducing the rate of egg production and increasing the generation time. In this respect it

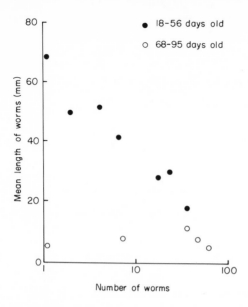

Fig. 25 Mean lengths of *Sobolevicanthus gracilis* in Mallard ducklings. (After Avery, 1969.)

enhances the crowding effects. The parasite population is further curtailed at high densities by the larval cestodes causing parasitic castration of the intermediate hosts and so reducing their population. Thus a series of feedback controls appear to operate upon this system to regulate the parasite population size.

A rather similar situation was found to occur amongst the hymenolepid cestodes of wild ducks in Poland by Wisniewski *et al.* (1958). The bulk of the parasites were small and stunted. Increasing crowding checked the growth and in some cases also the development and maturation of the cestodes. Competition and repeated invasion by juveniles could be excluded as causes, and it was again considered that this retardation was due to a reaction on the part of the host which rendered it less suitable for later infections. Death and loss of adults alleviated the effects of the factors checking growth and allowed some parasites to resume growth at a normal rate. Whatever the mechanism responsible, and there is no indication at all that it has an immunological basis, its effect was again to reduce the rate of parasite reproduction and increase the generation time, thereby slowing the build up of the parasite population.

PARASITES OF WILD GULLS

The infection levels and their changes of the parasites of herring gulls appears to be related primarily to both the diet and the behaviour of the birds (Threlfall, 1967). Crowding of birds in colonies at the time of breeding leads to increase in infection levels of parasites with a direct life cycle or with only one intermediate host such as the nematode *Cyathostoma lari*. The chicks become infected with such species first, due to the crowded conditions in the breeding colony favouring parasite transmission and the chicks' habit of feeding around the nest area. As they move farther away to feed, the levels of infection in these species decline with the decrease in probability of infection, and the birds acquire more species with indirect life cycles. For the first two months after leaving the colony they feed extensively upon fish, and so acquire digeneans such as *Cryptocotyle lingua* which utilise marine hosts. The occurrence of this parasite in older birds is almost confined to winter, when they feed extensively upon the shore line and upon fish and molluscs. In summer, by contrast, when gulls feed inland they acquire completely different parasites such as *C. lari* and other species which use terrestrial animals as their intermediate hosts. The incidence and infection levels of the marine species decline during this period as re-infection of the gulls is not possible.

A similar situation was found by Bakke (1972) in his studies of the parasites of the common gull. The birds arrived at the nesting site in April, nested in May, produced chicks in July and left again in September. Their parasite fauna could be divided into three groups depending upon the habits of the intermediate hosts, and the infection levels reflected directly the diet, both qualitative and quantitative, of the gulls. The overall incidence and levels of infection increased after arrival at the nesting site to reach a peak in July, but the composition of the parasite fauna changed throughout the period. On arrival, following marine feeding, the infection comprised mainly the marine species such as *Cryptocotyle*. These species persisted all through the breeding season, and even increased in incidence. In May, however, the gulls acquired several additional species that were present only in the breeding area and which employed terrestrial intermediate hosts, such as *Leucochloridium*. The levels of many of these declined later in the season. Other species such as *Tylodelphys* sp. became abundant only in August, when the birds fed extensively upon freshwater fish. Thus, the majority of parasites exhibited seasonal cycles in incidence and intensity of infection which could be related directly to the feeding behaviour of the gulls.

REGULATION OF PARASITE INFECTION LEVELS IN BIRDS

It is clear that many parasites of domestic birds provoke host responses when their density rises above certain levels, and that the parasite populations are regulated to some extent at least by these responses. The regulation may involve immune responses, changes in the suitability of the host not having an immunological basis, and intra-specific competition amongst the parasites. All the methods are supplementary and can and do function as negative feedback controls upon infection levels. It is far from clear, however, whether these methods are employed and are effective under natural conditions and in wild birds.

The conditions under which domestic birds are kept are conducive to the build up of heavy parasitic infections, especially of species of protozoans and nematodes having a direct life cycle. It seems clear that natural populations of cestodes in ducks are also subject to some forms of feedback controls, but the studies on gulls suggest that infection levels are dependent upon host dietary changes and other ecological factors rather than upon host responses. The ability of birds to develop resistance to low level infections of protozoans would suggest, however, that host responses could play some part in the regulation of wild bird parasites. It may well be therefore that parasite levels in wild birds are for the most part kept at low levels by the low probabilities of infection and by changes in host ecology, possibly aided by host responses. When infection levels rise, then responses may play a more important part in regulation. This may seldom, if ever, happen amongst gulls, since their changes in feeding habits restrict the time when conditions are favourable for the transmission of the parasite. It may only occur at certain times of year amongst ducks, when they aggregate in large numbers for feeding in winter and breeding in summer and conditions for parasite transmission are exceptionally favourable. It may occur at all times of year amongst domestic birds, which are kept at high densities for economic reasons. Under most natural conditions therefore bird-parasite systems are probably controlled in a similar manner to those of fish, but it is clear that host responses can play a far more important part in effecting feedback regulation than they do amongst fish parasites. Bird-parasite systems, for these reasons, must be considered to be inherently more stable.

9 Population changes within mammal definitive hosts

PROTOZOAN PARASITES OF MAMMALS

Most, if not all, protozoan parasites of mammals elicit specific responses by their hosts. In general the conditions for the responses and their manifestations are similar to those of bird parasites (p. 106). The effects upon the parasites are variable, ranging from inhibition of reproduction through agglutination and lysis to phagocytosis of the protozoans, and protection against re-infection may not be complete. It appears that a residual infection may often persist at a low level in a host, maintaining a state of immunity which lasts only whilst the parasites persist in the hosts known as premunition. In general, therefore, most protozoan-mammal systems are in a state of rather unstable equilibrium between infectivity of the parasite and its virulence, and the strength and effectiveness of the host response.

MAMMALIAN TRYPANOSOMES

The way in which infection levels of protozoans can be regulated by host responses is shown clearly by infections of *Trypanosoma lewisi* in rats (Taliafero, 1932). After an incubation period, the length of which depends upon the size of the initial infection, the parasites appear in the blood and start to reproduce, and the level of infection rises. About 10 days after infection the rat produces an ablastin antibody which prevents the trypanosomes undergoing further division but does not kill them. When reproduction has virtually ceased, another antibody is produced which kills the division forms only and causes the level of infection to decline (Fig. 26). The adults surviving are resistant to this antibody, but cannot reproduce and so build up the infection due to the continuing presence of the ablastin. They persist for about another month, when the production of a second trypanocidal antibody kills all the trypanosomes and eliminates the infection. The rats then exhibit a life long immunity to re-infection. The trypanosomes that survive the first antibody are still infective to fleas, so completion of the life cycle and transmission is still possible for as long as they remain in the rat.

Populations of other trypanosome species behave in a very different manner (Desowitz, 1970). Infections of mammals with trypanosomes of the *brucei* group, including *T. brucei, T. rhodesiense* and *T. gambiense,* undergo cyclical rise and falls in level (Fig. 27). These changes are associated with changes in both the structure and antigenicity of the parasites. During the rise in infection level or parasitaemia the slender form of the parasite predominates, and during the fall, the stumpy form (Vickerman, 1971). The stumpy form is infective to the vector

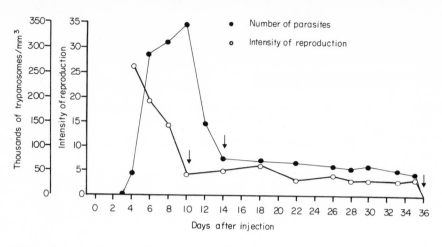

Fig. 26 The normal course of infection with *Trypanosoma lewisi* in the blood of a rat. The arrows indicate the times of the three primary manifestations of host immunity. (After Alesandro, 1970.)

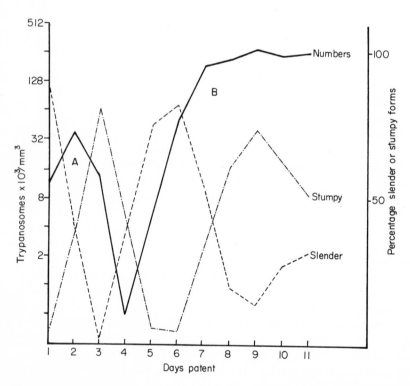

Fig. 27 Relationships between the course of infection and variations in trypanosome morphology for a strain of *T. brucei rhodesiense* in a rat. The populations at A and B belong to different serotypes. (After Vickerman, 1971.)

and the slender form to mammals. Loss of ability to produce stumpy forms is associated with loss of ability to infect flies, but does not interfere with changes in antigenicity. In the course of an infection, the trypanosomes undergo antigenic variation. The antigens occur in a predictable sequence and none occurs twice. Twenty-two variants have been reported from *T. brucei* and 23 from *T. gambiense,* but the number may be unlimited. Each induces formation of a specific host antibody, effective only against that serotype, and on infecting a fly they revert to the parent type. The transformation from slender to stumpy form and the change from one serotype to another are probably induced by the host response.

The infection thus consists intially of slender forms, and the level rises until host antibodies are produced. Many of the parasites are then killed, and the infection level falls. The survivors, however, change to the stumpy form and to a different serotype. The infection then builds up again until antibodies to the new serotype are produced, when the whole cycle is repeated. The trypanosome population is able to survive and avoid the immune response it provokes since each parasite carries a full range of antigens, and some can switch to an alternative. The infection is thus never eliminated, but it may be reduced. It may persist for years as a chronic infection, as does *T. gambiense,* or for a few months only when, as with *T. rhodesiense,* the parasite is virulent and toxic and proves rapidly fatal.

Both natural resistance and host condition are also involved in limiting trypanosome infections. Adult Zebu cattle from West Africa may die of heavy *T. vivax* infections, but survive light ones if the grazing is good. Usually infection results in a series of acute parasitaemias, followed by a low level of infection. The pattern of events corresponds with the immunological changes in the host, the antibody level rising during the rise, and falling with the fall. Shorthorn cattle, however, are generally fairly resistant to *T. vivax* unless suffering nutritional deprivation or disease (Desowitz, 1970). Infection results in a low parasitaemia and a high level of antibodies. However, calves from immune dams in a tsetse fly free area are only partially immune, and if removed from trypanosomes for several generations are completely susceptible to infection. Control of infections therefore involves hereditary factors and not just antibodies, and it is not at all certain that infections in ungulates are regulated by immune responses.

This appears also to be the case with infections of *T. cruzi.* Some natural resistance occurs, especially in endemic areas, and some partial immunity may occur in cattle, especially if exposure to the parasite is continuous (Goble, 1970). This immunity may wane if exposure to the parasite ceases. Humans may also become immune to infection with *Leishmania tropica* following spontaneous healing of lesions (Stauber, 1970). The lesion must, however, go through the full cycle of natural changes, and if the sore is removed before spontaneous recovery is complete, no immunity develops. The immunity does not appear to be related to antibody production or to serological changes. *L. donovani* is, however, almost always fatal. The host does respond by producing antibodies, but due probably to the location of the parasite in the reticulo-endothelial system, these are ineffective. Thus, responses to flagellates may limit the level of infection, but more often antibodies do not appear to be very effective either because of the site of the parasite or its ability to avoid them. It would appear that whilst acquired immunity may regulate rat trypanosomes, it may only play a small part in controlling many other flagellates.

MAMMALIAN MALARIAS

Many rodent malarias provoke effective immune responses by their hosts (Zuckerman, 1970). Infections of *Plasmodium berghei* in rats and *P. chabaudi* in mice rise to a high level and then decline. The decline is accompanied by an increase in antibody production. A low level of infection then persists, causing a state of premunition and the host becomes immune to re-infection. *P. vinckei* in mice is usually fatal, but if natural cure takes place or if the infection is terminated by drugs, the hosts become immune. Rodents in general appear to exhibit true immunity to the same strain of malaria, which is most effective against the schizont and merozoite stages. In many cases, however, correlation with serological changes is weak, and the lymphatic system is undoubtedly involved to a considerable extent.

The responses of primates to species of *Plasmodium* are more variable, and all stages of effectiveness may occur from complete immunity to re-infection to little or no immunity when the infection terminates fatally (Garnham, 1970). The situation is very complex, as some parasites show some antigenic variation and the degree of immunity shown depends upon the strain of both host and parasite. Natural resistance plays some part, and both circulating antibodies and the lymph-macrophage systems, especially phagocytes, are involved. Antibodies are produced by humans in response to *P. vivax, P. malariae* and *P. falciparum,* and are effective against the parasites but seldom cause their elimination. They attack and eliminate most of the erythrocytic schizonts, but this results in a latent infection since some survive and/or the exo-erythrocytic stage persists in the liver (except for *P. falciparum*). When the antibody level falls, or when the antigenicity of the parasite changes, the infection level increases again. The parasites may thus persist in the hosts for years if they do not cause fatal infections, causing cycles of infection and recovery until the stages in the liver die out, and in endemic areas hosts generally only exhibit incomplete immunity. Where the parasite is virulent, as with *P. knowlesi* in rhesus monkeys, the infection level rises unchecked, and the parasite kills the host before any protective mechanism can be employed against it. True immunity may result when primates are infected by unusual species of *Plasmodium,* and the initial infection is also limited. An intermediate situation is found in infections of oriental macaques with *P. inui.* The infection level starts to rise, but then is checked and remains at a low level as the host immune system becomes operative. This destroys most, though not all, of the parasites, and whilst these persist new infections are eliminated and so the parasites persist for long periods.

It is clearly impossible to generalise about malarial infections. The most that can be said is that many mammal hosts can reduce infection levels to some extent, and that this involves both natural and acquired resistance, but the effectiveness varies from system to system, and many malarias can avoid the responses and persist for long periods. Their incidence will still depend to a large extent on the habits of their vectors.

DIGENEAN PARASITES OF MAMMALS

NATURAL INFECTIONS

Amongst the digeneans of mammals, *Fasciola* and the schistosomes have attracted most attention. The situation with respect to regulation of *Fasciola* is still far from clear (Dawes and Hughes, 1964). Some hosts show natural resistance, in some a tissue response confers some resistance to re-infection, and in some there appears to be no host response and infection levels are determined by the number of metacercariae ingested.

The responses of hosts to schistosome infections are also very variable, and it is again difficult to distinguish in some cases between natural and acquired immunity (Lewert, 1970; Smithers and Terry, 1969; Stirewelt, 1963). Field data on human populations indicates the existence of some degree of acquired immunity. People are able to live in areas of countries such as Egypt where they are under continual re-exposure to infection. The symptoms of schistosomiasis are less severe in older persons, and in many parts of the world it is essentially a disease of young people. This cannot be due just to age immunity since adults are susceptible on encountering infections for the first time. They do not, however, provide conclusive evidence for acquired immunity, since the manifestations could be due to enhanced natural immunity resulting from exposure.

EXPERIMENTAL INFECTIONS

Numerous laboratory studies have been carried out using a variety of schistosomes and hosts, and a reduction in the proportion of parasites reaching the portal veins, stunting and early death when compared with controls have been accepted as criteria of acquired immunity (Table 53). Infections of mice

Table 53 Status of resistance to challenge infections with some schistosomes. (From Stirewelt, 1963.)

Host	Schistosome species	Criteria of resistances: reduced
Man	*haematobium*	Number of eggs: disease
Rhesus monkey	*mansoni*	Number of eggs
,,	*japonicum*	Number of eggs
,,	*douthitti*	Number of worms: disease
Mouse	*douthitti*	Number and size of worms
,,	*mansoni*	Number of worms
,,	*japonicum*	Number of worms

and rhesus monkeys with *S. douthitti* show that in some cases immunised animals harbour fewer adults, and that these are stunted and retarded in development. A primary infection of males only can immunise the host against subsequent infection by males, but not by females. A primary infection by females can confer partial immunity to males, females, or bisexual infections. In other cases, however, no immunity could be demonstrated. Some degree of immunity could also be induced by *S. haematobium*. Egg production declined and eventually ceased in infections of Macaca monkeys, and no eggs appeared after a second infection. Children may also show complete resistance to re-infection by *S. haematobium* after treatment for an initial infection, although in other cases only reduced establishment of the parasite was apparent. Establishment of a secondary infection of *S. japonicum* in mice and hamsters may be reduced to around 40%, and some species of monkeys and rabbits also show some acquired immunity to this species. Small regular infections and large single infections appear to give similar results, and it is not at all certain that enhanced natural immunity is not in some measure responsible for these effects. In rhesus monkeys, however, primary infections of *S. japonicum* can confer almost complete immunity to re-infection. Protection may last for from one to three years, but is rarely absolute in the absence of a latent infection. In some instances *S. mansoni* can also induce immunity. Secondary infections of mice and hamsters may show from 19% to 99% reduction in establishment. Resistance to re-infection usually increases with age. In most primates immunity is manifested by a decrease in egg production in a second infection and by the ability of the host to tolerate a lethal dose.

CONCOMITANT IMMUNITY

In rhesus monkeys, infections of *S. mansoni* produce eggs after six weeks, the rate of production increases from 8–12 weeks and then falls, but persists at a steady level. Light infections undoubtedly persist at low levels for long periods, but resistance to re-infection also occurs. This is complete after 21 weeks, and partial at 3 weeks. Transfer of *S. mansoni* from other hosts to rhesus monkeys protected the monkeys against new cercarial infections, thus clearly demonstrating the existence of immunity. The adults that had been transferred, however, maintained a steady rate of egg production and were evidently able to avoid the immune response that they themselves provoked.

This condition, known as concomitant immunity, has been studied in detail by Smithers and Terry (1968) and Smithers (1968). Adult worms transferred from mice, hamsters and monkeys into monkeys all induce the same order of immunity, but their behaviour in the new host differs. In parasites transferred from monkeys eggs appear quickly and soon reach a high level of production; in parasites from mice egg production is initially checked, then after 4–6 weeks rises to a comparable level, whereas in worms from hamsters few if any eggs are laid. This suggests that worms from mice, though not from hamsters, are able to adapt in some way to their hosts. Adults were then grown in mice and transplanted to new monkeys immunised against *mice* (Fig. 28). Here they were destroyed, and behaved like ham-

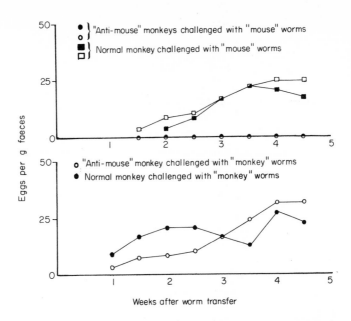

Fig. 28 Egg counts of *Schistosoma mansoni* in normal monkeys and monkeys immunised against mouse liver and spleen, to which pairs of 'mouse' or 'monkey' worms were transferred. (After Smithers, 1968.)

ster worms transplanted to monkeys. Clearly it is possible to immunise monkeys against mouse worms by using mouse, not parasite, antigens, and this indicates that mouse antigens are present on mouse worms. These must be acquired gradually, since all flukes from mice after 15 days infection possess them, whereas only some do after 7 days, and cercariae do not possess them at all. It is suggested therefore that *S. mansoni* adapts to the rhesus monkey by acquiring host antigens and thus disguising themselves as host tissue and thereby avoiding the immune responses they provoke. This theory contrasts strongly with the ideas of reduced antigenic disparity between parasite and host and molecular mimicry advanced by Dineen (1963) and Damian (1964), which suggest genotypic rather than phenotypic adaptation to the host.

It appears therefore that schistosomes can induce some degree of resistance to re-infection in most hosts, but the appearance of resistance is erratic and depends upon the conditions of the experiment, the experimental procedure, the duration of the infection and the strain of host and parasite. In some systems resistance may be completely absent, or its development may be very gradual and take years. The demonstration of antibodies in association with protection is also elusive and depends on the conditions. Raised immunoglobulin levels are characteristic of infections, but resistance may also be due to enhancement of innate mechanisms such as skin thickening. Furthermore, immunity, when manifested, many be of the concomitant type. Thus, the level of most schistosome infections is probably depressed to some extent by host responses, but this will vary in different host-parasite systems and under different conditions. In very few cases are the parasites completely eliminated. The exhibition of both partial and concomitant immunity ensures that some of the parasites survive and reproduce. The incidence of infection in a host population is governed by the ecological factors that determine the degree of contact between the host and parasite (pp. 134, 136–138), and the probability of infection is generally very low (Table 4). Where immunity is not strongly manifested, these same ecological factors will also determine the level of infection in most individual hosts, which will relate to the frequency with which they make contact with cercariae.

ADULT CESTODE PARASITES IN MAMMALS

Whereas the majority of cestode larvae in mammals are able to produce strong and effective host immune responses, the majority of adults are not (Weinmann, 1966, 1970). They are often immunogenic, but the antibodies produced are ineffective against the cestode. Thus *Hymenolepis microstoma* can induce antibody formation in its normal host, the mouse, but the antibodies have no effect on the parasite (Moss, 1971). In contrast, the antibodies it provokes in rats prevent its growth and reproduction. Following an initial infection of sheep with *Moniezia* there is a decrease in survival of parasites in later infections, an extension of the development period and a depression of the reproductive rate. These effects are more noticeable in older sheep, but cannot be correlated with antibody or other serological changes.

Only in infections of mice with *H. nana* has a host response capable of reducing the level of infection and involving immune systems been clearly demonstrated. This species may undergo a direct life cycle in a single host individual by autoinfection, and the cysticercoid, when in the mouse tissue, is strongly antigenic. Effective immunity and regulation has only been demonstrated in the direct cycle, since it requires the presence of the cysticercoid in the host tissue and not just in the intestine lumen. Autoinfection leads to a massive rise in infection level due to the appearance of the second generation of parasites, but thereafter immunity to further autoinfestation or to re-infection develops. Larvae of the new infection are unable to invade the mucosa of previously infected hosts and so cannot transform into cysticercoids. Immune serum may also confer protection against the invasive stage, but not against eggs or cysts. The resulting immunity may be absolute and may persist after removal of the parasites that provoked it.

Amongst most cestodes, however, host diet and condition, and especially stress, and intra-specific competition amongst the parasites are the more important controls on infection levels. The presence of one or a few cestodes of an initial infection may reduce the rate of establishment in later infections, a phenomenon known often as premunition and exhibited by *H. diminuta* in rats and *Taenia saginata* in man amongst other species. Inhibition of development in this case relates to the original worm burden, and does not involve antibody production or any immunological response. There is evidence in *H. diminuta* at least to suggest that it is a manifestation of intra-specific competition (Roberts, 1961) or due to the later infections being unable to occupy the most favourable site. Thus, with the exception of *H. nana,* tapeworm-mammal definitive host systems are not regulated by host responses, and the major regulatory factor is intra-specific competition amongst the parasites affecting level of infection, whilst incidence depends on contact with infective larvae.

NEMATODE PARASITES OF MAMMALS

GENERAL CONSIDERATIONS

The majority of studies on nematode populations have been carried out on strongyles infecting farm animals and rodents. The conditions under which the farm animals live are far from natural and are often conducive to the build up of large parasite populations. Conclusions derived from such studies may therefore not be generally applicable to nematode populations under natural field conditions. These species all have direct life cycles, and their high fecundity is offset by heavy mortality amongst free living stages due to climatic factors. Small changes in climate may have very large effects upon the parasite population: if only in 1 in 1000 larvae survive on the pastures then a decrease in mortality in the region of only 1% may lead to an increase of up to 900% in some species. Since development rate is also affected by climate, infection of hosts is frequently seasonal although egg production may be continuous.

Resistance to infection by the hosts has several manifestations, one or several of which may be apparent or predominant in any particular host-parasite system. Where several are evidenced, they may appear in sequence depending either on increasing infection level or on time of year. Furthermore, resistance is often only manifested at all above a particular threshold level of infection. This level may be lowered in second and subsequent infections. Thus a wide variety of host responses and climatic effects can operate upon the parasites, and these may and do change from habitat to habitat.

NIPPOSTRONGYLUS IN RATS

The mechanism of regulation of infection levels of *Nippostrongylus brasiliensis* in the laboratory rat has been studied in some detail (Ogilvie and Jones, 1971). Four stages can be recognised in the course of a single primary heavy infection (Fig. 29). According to Jarrett *et al.* (1968) between 40 and 60% of the infective larvae are lost in the course of migration to the intestine (Loss phase 1). The size of the adult population then remains constant (plateau phase) and eggs are produced from day 6. On day 12 expulsion of adults begins and continues at an exponential rate (loss phase 2), although a small residual population remains. These are mainly males, and live in the duodenum and not in the preferred site, the jejunum. The rats are now partly resistant to re-infection, and in

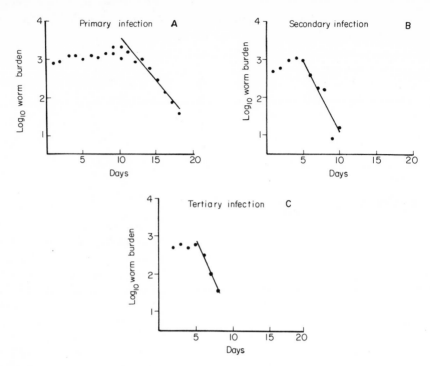

Fig. 29 The survival of *Nippostrongylus brasiliensis* in experimental infections of rats. (After Jarrett *et al.*, 1968.)

subsequent infections a lower proportion of adults establish, the plateau phase is shorter, expulsion is faster and the development of some larvae is retarded at the fourth larval stage. The adults also inhabit a different region of the intestine.

In small initial infections there is a gradual loss of parasites over 30 days, and if the population is allowed to build up gradually by continued exposure to small numbers elimination is not drastic. The infection level is reduced in all instances to a threshold level of about 40 worms. Neonatal or new born rats exposed to infections of 200–250 larvae permit the parasite population to persist, and it declines slowly. If exposed to over 250 larvae, expulsion takes place later (day 17), ceases at a threshold of 200 adults, and persists into the adult life of the rat. In subsequent infections, if the initial infection is not rejected it behaves as a primary infection: if it is it behaves as a subsequent or secondary infection. Reinfection before 7 weeks results in an adult parasite population at the neonatal threshold, and after 7 weeks at the adult rat threshold.

The response thus depends on the age of the rat, the response to the initial infection and the size of both infecting doses. Reduced infectivity and reproductive rate of the initial population and its survivors, the residual population, is due to an immune response, not to parasite senescence, as can be shown by transfer experiments, and expulsion of secondary infections can be prevented by immunosuppressin drugs. Parasites in a secondary infection are less immunogenic, and can adapt to the immune host to some extent. The host response involves both the production of antibodies, which damage the parasites, and an inflammatory response which causes expulsion. Thus, rats are able to regulate their *N. brasiliensis* infections about a threshold level and prevent super-infection by employing their immune systems, although the threshold level is not constant but depends upon the age of the rat and the conditions of infection.

SHEEP NEMATODES

The levels of sheep nematode infections are also regulated to a large extent by 'self-cure' reactions involving the host immune response, although the seasonal changes in population size are due to the post-parturient rise (p. 25) and climatic influences (Crofton, 1963; Michel, 1969). For most of the year adult sheep are resistant to infection and maintain a low level of parasites, but this rises after parturition in spring (Fig. 30) due to a temporary relaxation in resistance associated with host endocrine changes. The rise occurs even when few inhibited larvae are present in the host and in sheep with no residual parasite population, and so is due in part to increased establishment of larvae ingested during the period of lactation, although it may also be due in part to resumption of development by inhibited larvae when these are present. Shortly after parturition the sheep resume their normal immune state, and the threshold for resistance returns to its normal level. The eggs from these sheep thus produce infective larvae at the time when lambs commence grazing. These and any remaining winter residue are acquired by the lambs, and the parasite population builds up rapidly in summer.

This increase may be exponential as a result of cycles of reinfection involving several generations, or may involve only one or two generations if auto-infestation is rare and the level of larvae on the pasture depends on eggs produced by ewes rather than by lambs. The parasite population level attained depends upon the success of hatching, the survival rate of the larvae on the pasture and the overall parasite generation time, and these are all dependent upon climatic conditions. In late summer, when lambs are 4–6 months old and their immune systems fully developed, the parasite population level falls abruptly due to a massive host reaction preventing new infections and to the increasingly unfavourable climatic conditions. Levels of infection in lambs then remain at the same level as in adult sheep.

Nematodirus battus behaves rather differently to the other species, as its eggs overwinter on the pasture, require spells of cold temperature before hatching and hatch in spring (Crofton, 1963). The level of infective larvae on the pastures in spring thus depends upon the population size in the previous year and the winter climate. Eggs produced by parasites in spring lambs cannot usually hatch out until they have experienced the cold temperatures of the following winter. If, however, they do hatch out in the same year due to cold autumn temperatures, the lambs have by then attained a state of immunity and infection is not possible. Thus this species does not undergo cycles of autoinfestation, and transmission is largely from one generation of lambs to another. For most other species the

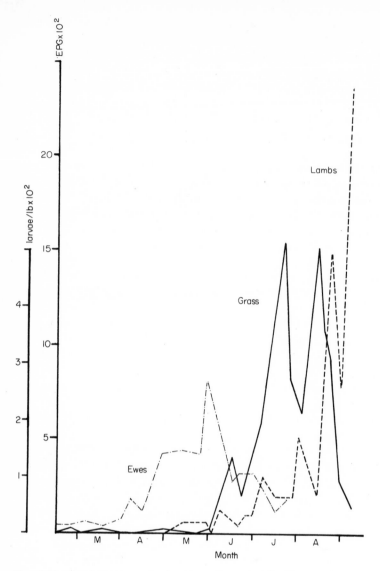

Fig. 30 The faecal egg counts of ewes and their lambs and the herbage infestations (chiefly *Ostertagia* spp. and *Trichostrongylus* spp.) on the pasture which they grazed. (After Michel, 1969.)

period of infestation is short due to climate and host resistance, and infection levels can be regulated by self-cure.

Although self-cure involves both circulating antibodies and hypersensitivity responses in all species, its mechanisms and thresholds vary between host-parasite systems. Self-cure in *Haemonchus contortus* is never complete. Resistance is related to re-infection, and if this occurs immediately after the primary infection or does not occur at all, then there is no self-cure. Expulsion of parasites is

126

considered to require a challenge infection, although some recent work (Allanby and Urquart, 1973) has suggested that under some conditions self-cure occurs in the absence of re-infection and is not immunological in nature. Following a secondary infection, the original infection is lost as a result of the self-cure but the secondary infection establishes. In a series of experimental infections Dineen and his colleagues (Dineen *et al.*, 1965; Donald *et al.*, 1969; Wagland and Dineen, 1967) were able to demonstrate that host responses only controlled the infection level when it exceeded a threshold value (Fig. 31). Self-cure was an extreme response to repeated heavy infections, and lighter repeated infections were controlled to a large extent by retardation of larval development at the fourth larval stage. Infections below the threshold level produced no effects independent of the host response, but continuous exposure above it provoked increasingly stronger responses. Repeated very heavy infections could lead to a state of host immunological exhaustion, where infections were tolerated.

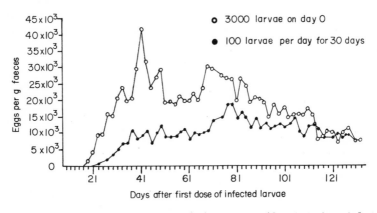

Fig. 31 Mean faecal egg counts for *Haemonchus contortus* following primary infections in sheep. (After Dineen *et al.*, 1965.)

The *H. contortus*-sheep system has also been studied in detail by Whitlock and his colleagues (Whitlock, 1966; Ratcliffe *et al.*, 1969). Their analysis of this interaction is discussed in detail later (p. 139), but they agree that populations of *H. contortus* are regulated. They consider that at the level of nematodes and individual sheep the course of infection is difficult to predict, but at the level of host and parasite populations the course of an infection is predictable to a high degree of precision. They consider that such a level of homeostasis can only be achieved by regulation of *all* the parasite's activities, including development rate and egg production, and they propose a systems model for such regulation (p. 139). They later (Whitlock *et al.*, 1972) go on to consider the time dependency of this system in more detail. They suggest that there are host-mediated factors common to and capable of regulating the parameters of mixed strongyle infections, and that there is some device capable of resource allocation. To account for the time dependency of control they propose three hypotheses; that through the action of biological clocks, the parent parasites in each annual cycle are able to programme the rate of development through each generation; that the rate of development of the parasites is related to the rate of senescence and death; and that the rate of development and death for each individual nematode is set at the start of each season by a host factor acting upon the parasite. Further testing of these hypotheses may contribute greatly to understanding the dynamics of this host-parasite system.

OSTERTAGIA IN CALVES

Regulation of infection levels of *Ostertagia ostertagi* in calves appears to be achieved by a rather different mechansim, and one, according to Michel (1969, 1970), not involving a threshold or a dramatic expulsion of parasites. Daily infection of calves results in an increasing proportion of the infective dose being retarded at the early fourth larval stage. Removal of the adult parasites by drugs stimulates these larvae to resume development and replace the lost adults. The calves remain susceptible to infection (Fig. 32) and continued infection reduces the rate at which the level of inhibited larvae decreases. Thus the loss of adults stimulates the resumption of development, and they are replaced from the

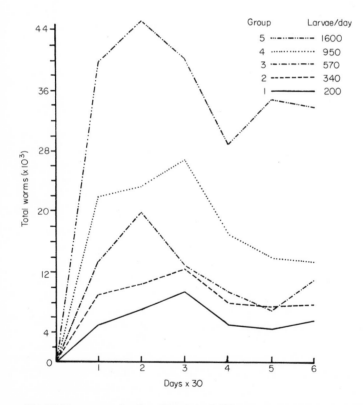

Fig. 32 Mean worm burdens (fourth and fifth stage) of *Ostertagia ostertagi* in groups of calves experiencing different daily infection regimes. (After Michel, 1970.)

128

reservoir of arrested larvae. Under natural conditions, the loss of adults is exponential and the rate is proportional to the number of adults present. This in turn is proportional to the infection rate, so loss of worms is directly related to infection levels and recruitment rate.

Exposure to new infections at a constant rate, therefore, would result in a parasite infection in a state of equilibrium where loss and gain of parasites are equal. The population in the intestine would be maintained at the level at which the new infection stopped, and loss is in no way related to a threshold level. Since lost adults are replaced by larvae resuming development, there is a constant turnover of parasites through the population. This turnover is slower at lower infection rates, when a smaller proportion of the larvae are inhibited, and increasing resistance is experienced as the level of infection rises.

The rate of egg production is regulated by a separate self-contained mechanism and is restricted to a steady level by the host, not by the number of mature females. Immunosuppressin drugs raise the level of egg output, but do not affect larval inhibition, and even when antibody level falls to a tenth of its usual level the parasite population size remains constant. The total number of eggs produced by a calf is the same whether it is given a single dose of larvae or repeated doses, and is similar in calves with different parasite burdens. Thus populations of *O. ostertagi* are controlled by at least two independent mechanisms, one of which regulates the rate of egg production and the other of which regulates infection levels by relating loss, gain and replacement of adult parasites. Both function in a feedback manner to stabilise the system.

The level of infestation of *O. ostertagi* on pastures depends more on climate than on rate of contamination. Resistance develops slowly in calves, so that they are not resistant for the whole of their first grazing season. The majority of larvae ingested in their first autumn become inhibited in development, and this serves to carry the infection from year to year. Overwintering larvae originate from eggs produced before June, and their residue are acquired by autumn born calves in spring. They mature, and their progeny appear on the pasture in July. The calf becomes re-infected by these and the parasite population level rises. The eggs of this generation produce larvae on the herbage in September, and these, if ingested, are inhibited. Calves enter their second year with a residual population composed of those acquired in July and those in September. Thereafter resistance develops, and there is a turnover of parasites as described above. The population changes and their regulation mechanisms thus differ from those of sheep nematodes.

STABILITY OF MAMMALIAN HOST-PARASITE SYSTEMS

Mammals clearly differ from poikilotherm hosts in their much greater ability to respond to the parasites, and most are able to regulate the levels of parasitic infections to some extent. The mechanism of the response and its effectiveness, however, vary from system to system. Host immune responses may be the only control upon parasite numbers, but frequently other independent controls also operate, including competition. Nearly all these controls function in a negative feedback manner, and will tend to stabilise the system.

Despite this inherent stability, parasite populations are still liable to large fluctuations because of their dependence upon climatic factors. This may act as an additional control upon population increase, though not a feedback one, when conditions are unfavourable because of the heavy mortality encountered in the free living stages. This dependence upon climate, however, also allows populations to increase and take full advantage of favourable conditions. Such increases can then only be checked by host responses and the return of unfavourable conditions. Climate thus has a pronounced influence upon the incidence of infection within the host population, whereas host responses govern the levels of infection within the hosts and introduce stability.

It is of importance to the perpetuation of the system that the responses control, rather than eliminate, the parasites, and that a proportion of the parasite population is able to avoid the harmful response it provokes, whether by antigenic variation, concomitant immunity or the necessity for a threshold to provoke a response at all. By these mechanisms only the surplus population is eliminated and infection levels are kept to a level at which they do the minimum damage to the hosts. This ensures the survival of the parasite population and the continued existence of the host-parasite system. The achievement of homeostasis by the mammals themselves is thus paralleled by the achievement of a high degree of homeostasis by their host-parasite systems.

10 Epidemiology and models of host-parasite systems

FOCAL NATURE OF PARASITIC INFECTIONS

The last few chapters of this book have been concerned with the identification and estimation of the relative importance of the factors that control the infection levels of parasites within their hosts, and so their population sizes. For the sake of convenience intermediate and definitive host-parasite systems have largely been considered independently, but of course changes in infection levels in each host and changes in each system are to a large degree interdependent, since the controls operating on each system will influence the parasite population as a whole.

It has also been suggested that many host-parasite systems are inherently unstable, and that infection levels depend upon local host behaviour and habitat conditions. Even where the systems are inherently stable, and feedback controls operate, the parasites are dependent upon climate and levels of infection may be governed principally by climatic conditions and by ecological conditions that influence the success of transmission from one host to another. It follows therefore that the size of, and changes in, any parasite population is closely related to the climatic and biotic conditions prevailing in the particular locality in which the parasite is living. Since these conditions change from locality to locality, and from time to time within a locality, the conditions favouring the parasite and hence its distribution may also be very local in both space and time.

Thus, although parasites may occur over wide areas of territory, their distribution is seldom homogeneous. Instead, they tend to be found in foci, in local areas where conditions favour their dissemination and survival. The foci may be discrete, and the distribution discontinuous, or some degree of spatial continuity may exist in which case foci of abundance can often be recognised. In either case, there is no reason to assume that the patterns of population change in each focus will be similar: indeed, if conditions differ between foci, then it would be expected that levels of infection and the patterns of population changes will also differ.

The focal nature of infections is particularly evident in parasites with aquatic stages in their life cycles, since each population must perforce be centred around a water body. Thus schistosomiasis is always related to water, and especially to still water and shaded conditions, since this is the situation preferred by its molluscan host and to which its definitive host is attracted. In an extreme situation, in the Yemen, the foci of infection were the mosques, since the pools provided next to them for ritual purposes were not only the only suitable sites in the area for the snails, but also sites to which the majority of humans were attracted, and in which, moreover, they had to make close contact with the snails by washing themselves for ritual purposes (Kuntz, 1952). By contrast *Onchocerca* is centred around rivers, especially fast flowing ones, since the larvae of its vector prefer almost torrential conditions. The creation of dams along rivers for hydro-electrical purposes in Africa may often have the dual consequence of extending the range and creating a new focus for schistosomes in the still conditions above the dam, whilst decreasing the vector population of *Onchocerca* above the dam but increasing it below and thus causing a shift in the focus of infection.

The location of disease foci may also depend upon host behavioural factors. Trypanosomiasis is a typically focal disease. Its level depends upon the interplay of parasite strain and virulence and host immunity, and, perhaps above all, the behaviour of the vector. The population of *T. gambiense* starts to increase in a locality when a population of tsetse flies becomes progressively anthrophilic and concentrates its biting activities upon man. The extent to which it does this depends upon the extent to which the human population is aggregated and the availability of alternative hosts for the flies. The relationship between parasite foci and human behaviour patterns has been discussed by Nelson (1972), and may be seen also in *Onchocerca*. On settlement of a human population near a river, the incidence of *O. volvulus* starts to increase due to the close proximity of man and vector. The flies become progressively more anthropophillic and infection levels rise still further. When the incidence of parasite induced blindness is high enough to seriously impair the activities of the human population, it moves to a new area. With this move, incidence of disease diminishes at first, but later starts to rise again and the cycle recommences, but the focus of the disease has moved.

EPIDEMIOLOGY OF PARASITES

Because parasite infections are focal in nature and because their population levels are so closely related to the conditions pertaining in each focus, it is often possible in a general way to relate the transmission and nature of infection to particular habitat types and landscapes. Thus, the level of mosquito-transmitted diseases such as malaria in any locality depends to a very great extent upon host choice and selection by the vector (Gillies, 1972). Some genera such as *Aedes* feed on a very wide range of animals, and choice is largely determined by ecological factors and host availability. Other genera show preferences for particular species or groups of species. Both host odour and ecology and mosquito flight patterns are important in influencing the degree of contact between vector and host, and so the level of the *Plasmodium* population. By considering both host and parasite behaviour, it is possible to recognise four sharply defined epidemiological situations (Table 54). The savannah/cultivated situation is typical of human malaria in some parts of the world, where mosquitoes breed at considerable distance from human settlements and have to disperse widely in order to make contact with man. Mortality amongst mosquitoes in the course of such flights is high, and intensity of parasite transmission often correspondingly

Table 54 Epidemiological situations in relation to movements of vectors and hosts. (From Gillies, 1972.)

Nidus	Savannah/ cultivated	Forest/ woodland	Urban/ domestic	Deep caves
Flight pattern of vector	Wide ranging ill defined ambit	Sharply defined ambit	Unrestricted short flights	Movement within single cavern
Movements of host	Static often indoors	Mobile	Mobile or static	Static within cave
Host attack released by:	Vector flying into host-stream	Host-stream impinging on resting or locally flying vector	Endogenous rhythm	Endogenous rhythm
Vector encounters with host stimuli	Sporadic	Sporadic	Frequent	Continuous
Examples	*Anopheles* & malaria in Africa	*Anopheles* human malaria in Neotropics	*C. fatigans* & *Wuchereria bancrofti*	*Anopheles bamoni* & bat malaria in Congo

low. In the forest/woodland situation dispersal of the mosquito is far more restricted, and the parasite is acquired by man penetrating into the forest, which may also be sporadic. The vector is more likely to feed normally upon some host resident in the forest. In the urban/domestic situation man and the mosquito live in the same area in close contact, and so intensity of transmission and infection levels are high.

The pattern of leishmaniasis also varies in different areas, depending to a large extent upon the habits of the local vector and the status of reservoir hosts (Lainson and Shaw, 1971). In India, *L. donovani* is entirely a human domestic disease and is transmitted from man to man by the vector, with no reservoir hosts involved. The parasite occurs in the peripheral blood and is thus available to the sandfly vector, which breeds in association with man. It is capable of short flights only, and the disease is essentially local, progresses to adjacent sites and may reach local epidemic proportions. This is basically similar to the urban/domestic situation of mosquito-borne diseases. In other countries the progress of the disease is different, since the parasite may not be common in the peripheral blood and so the infection rate of sandflies feeding on man is low. Different species of vector may also be used which are not so closely associated with man, and reservoir hosts are incorporated into the life cycle. In such cases the disease may be chronic in the reservoir host and be transmitted only occasionally to man. Dogs generally fill this role, alone in the Mediterranean region, in association with rodents in East Africa and together with wild foxes in Brazil. In Peru *L. brasiliensis* occurs in dogs and humans, seldom reaches epidemic levels and causes only a mild form of disease to which adults become immune. It is only a semi-domestic disease. In Yucatan it occurs in rodents, not

133

dogs, and humans. It is here a disease of low altitude rain forests, since transmission is by a strictly sylvatic sand fly species. The distribution of the vector is discontinuous and it often has no association with humans, and the disease is correspondingly local and spasmodic in occurrence. It is never associated with urban areas, and man becomes infected through entering the forest. Thus *Leishmania* has endemic foci, and its incidence is determined by the behaviour, especially the degree of anthropophilly, of the vector, the status of the reservoir host, the status of man as a host, and the extent to which the distribution of the three hosts are coincident. All these features differ in each focus to give a different pattern of spread and transmission.

Each focus of schistosomiasis also has its own peculiar features, depending upon the climatic conditions prevailing and the ecology of the human and snail populations (Wright, 1970). In the Rhodesian high veldt, transmission of the parasite is low in January and February during the rainy season, since many snails are washed away, the temperature is too low for them to breed and there is little human contact with water. Between March and May there is little rain, the water conditions are settled, temperatures are higher, children make more contact with the water and the transmission rate increases. In winter, between June and September, the low night temperatures prevent the snail breeding, there is no human contact with water and the transmission rate falls almost to zero. The highest rate of transmission occurs between October and December, when temperatures are high, water levels low, the snails concentrate and breed rapidly, and human contact with water is maximal. In the low veldt, by contrast, temperatures are higher at all times, and transmission takes place throughout the year.

Even where the climate is uniform, transmission patterns may differ in local communities. Three localities within 20 miles in Gambia show quite different patterns of disease. Schistosomiasis is very rare or absent in the valley tribes since the snail hosts are rare or absent from the valleys. In the plateau regions, landscape depressions become filled with water in the rainy season only. The snail host in this area is able to withstand desiccation in the dry season. The depressions form a social centre for the tribes, and transmission is thus seasonally intense at the time of the rains. Amongst a third tribe living near streams transmission is most intense in the dry season, since the snails are washed away in the wet season but breed as the water falls and reach their maximum abundance in the pools in summer.

MODELS OF HOST-PARASITE SYSTEMS

THE CONCEPT OF MODELS

The approach to an understanding of host-parasite systems and parasite population changes considered so far in this book has involved the recording of events in the field, the design of supporting experiments, and their interpretation. One of the great difficulties of this approach is that of recording and analysing the enormous number of factors that can influence parasite populations and so lead to the different patterns of population change in different areas. The very complexity of the situation has also made it very difficult to generalise about parasites, their epidemiology or their population changes, and so to make predictions about their population levels under any particular set of conditions.

Of recent years an alternative approach to the understanding of host-parasite systems has been developed, that of attempting to construct models of the systems. This approach has been dependent upon the development of computers, since this has been the only way in which the numerous variables and their interactions can be handled. It consists in essence of simulating a host-parasite system, frequently upon an analogue computer, and then using the simulated model to see how the various environmental factors can affect the parasite population. In some cases, it may even be used to predict population levels under particular conditions. It is important to distinguish this type of modelling, however, from that discussed by Smyth (1969). He was concerned with the use of parasites and host-parasite systems as tools or 'models' to provide a biological system to investigate, usually experimentally, a particular biological phenomenon. For example, yeast cells are widely used as models for biochemical studies, and Smyth himself was advocating the use of *Echinococcus* as a model for differentiation studies. This sort of study and model is quite different from the mathematical modelling of parasite systems.

Mathematical or computer modelling of parasite systems can be an extremely valuable method of analysing and so of understanding parasite systems. The very construction of a model summarises the information about the system, both in the most concise way and in a way that permits easy comparison with the same system under different conditions, or with other systems. If the model gives a good approximation to field results, it can be assumed that the system has been understood sufficiently well for the model to be constructed. If the approximation is not good, either some information is lacking, or the available information is incorrect or incomplete. Thus the attempts to build a model, whether successful or not, may increase understanding of the system. A model may also be very useful in stimulating ideas for further research, and ultimately a very good one may even be used predictively, to estimate parasite population levels under any given set of conditions. It may also be used to study the way in which different variables and their interactions may affect parasites, and so to study the whole structure of the host-parasite system and its environment in a way that cannot otherwise be done, because of the complexity of the biological situation, the scarcity of material or difficulties of experimentation or manipulation in the field. The model can be used and constructed either qualitatively or quantitatively, but should incorporate all the factors known to have a significant influence on the parasite.

There are also of course inherent dangers in model building. The adequacy of a model depends to a large extent upon the accuracy of the basic assumptions built into it, and it is essential that these are defined in terms relevant to the system studied. Biological systems are so complex, however, that some degree of simplification is necessary to construct the models at all, and the dividing line between simplification and over-simplification is not always clear. Over-simplification may well distort the system it is intended to simulate, and this may result in a model that bears little relationship to the natural system. This situation may also arise if some of the parameters used to construct the model have no real biological basis. In other cases, there may just be insufficient data available to construct the model, or the data may be inaccurate, or the interpretation of it be incorrect. Clearly the construction of an inaccurate model may confuse rather than clarify understanding, and may result in erroneous predictions. There may also be other difficulties which make the results subject to cautious interpretation, such as the use of deterministic models for stochastic processes. Finally, conclusions based on models are derived by analogy, and this should always be borne in mind. Nevertheless, providing they are used to aid understanding and as a source of ideas rather than as a fully accurate reproduction of a biological system, models can be of considerable value, especially in the field of host-parasite systems and their regulation and stability. This will be exemplified by reference to four models.

MODELS OF SCHISTOSOME POPULATIONS

The first really detailed and comprehensive attempt to model host-parasite systems mathematically was that of MacDonald (1957) on malaria. Having studied the epidemiology of the disease, MacDonald attempted to construct a model of it that could describe and predict the differences in epidemiology of malaria found in different disease foci. At that time much of the necessary data was incomplete, and the situation was a very complex one indeed so that the model was of limited value only. Later, MacDonald went on to consider schistosomes, and he was able (1965) to construct a qualitative model of schistosome infections, with particular reference to the relative significance of the factors affecting transmission and to the effectiveness of various control measures employed against the disease.

Schistosomes and most other helminths differ from *Plasmodium* in that immunity to the parasite is relatively low and superinfection is possible. Furthermore, whereas protozoans multiply with ease initially due to asexual reproduction until checked by immunity, schistosome reproduction is restricted initially when they are rare because of the low probability of individuals of two sexes meeting. The probability of pairing was therefore an important consideration, and could be calculated for different levels of infection. MacDonald assumed that infections were random, that each sex had an equal probability of infection, and that parasites were long lived and produced eggs continuously.

The number of eggs reaching water depended upon the host population, the parasite burden, the degree of pairing and the rate of egg production. The proportion carried to water, related to environmental and sanitary conditions, he represented by a contamination factor. The probability of miracidia infecting a snail, the density of the snail population, the number of susceptible snails, their life span, multiplication within the snail, and degree and duration of cercarial output were represented by a snail factor. The probability of cercariae encountering a mammal, their efficiency and the number of contacts were represented by an exposure factor. The probability of mating within the vertebrate host and the longevity of the parasites were represented by a longevity factor. Different values were then assigned to each of these factors, and the course of infection to equilibrium or extinction computed. Control factors could be examined by testing the effects of consequent reduction in each factor. The break point, determined equally by all four factors, was the minimum parasite level necessary to permit a bisexual infection to persist.

The course of a computed standard infection is shown in Fig. 33A. Doubling the size of the factors lowered the break point and so allowed the introduction of the infection to take place at lower parasite densities, otherwise a massive invasion was needed to start an infection if all the factors were low. Doubling the contamination factor alone had little effect on the endemic level since miracidia are always more numerous than snails.

Control aimed at reducing population equilibrium levels to the break point, below which positive feedback would occur resulting in extermination of the infection. Control therefore did not have to be 100% efficient and reduce the population to zero, but only to break point level. When each factor was reduced to one fifth (Fig. 33B), contamination again had no effect upon reducing the population level. The reduction of the snail and exposure factors reduced the parasite population, but it took ten years to reach its new equilibrium level. Reduction in longevity took only two years. None of these schemes led to equilibrium level approaching break point, and at this level, treatment of individual hosts, whilst of value to the recipients, had little effect on the parasite population. Reduction of longevity, by treatment, to one fifth followed by reduction of exposure (Fig. 33C) could prove effective, and at an exposure level of one tenth or lower the break point was reached.

Finally, four types of control of apparently similar value in that each reduced one of the factors to one fifteenth were compared. Increase in sanitation measures had no effect on the parasite population (Fig. 33D). Reduction of the snail population and control of entry to water took 20 years to eliminate the parasite, but the combined effect of reducing treatment factor to one fifth and complementary lessening of exposure to one third or of snails to one third eliminated infection in 4–5 years.

A single method of control, therefore, or diffuse unco-ordinated activities are of little use since they only ameliorate the infection. Sanitation methods are also of little value, although they may increase the success of other methods. Safe water supplies provide the best single control method, since it reduces both exposure and contamination, but both this and snail control are very slow on their own. Elimination of the parasite needs an intensive, well planned campaign, which is quite practicable in view of the focal nature of the disease, and a general improvement in public health. Thus, on the basis of just a qualitative model, MacDonald was able not only to indicate clearly the relative significance of the factors influencing schistosome population levels, but was also able to apply this information and make direct recommendations for

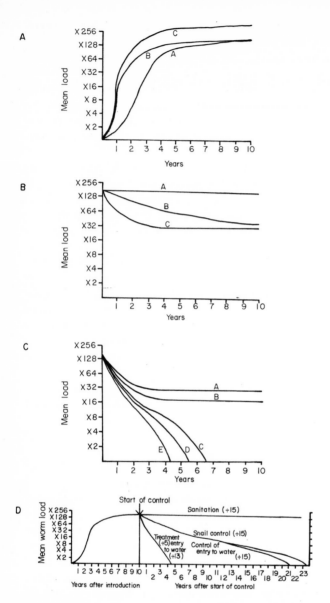

Fig. 33 Computer models of schistosome infections. A. The standard infection, A, and the curves expected following doubling the contamination factor, B, and either the snail or exposure factor, C.

B. The effect of control by modifying standard factors by, A, reducing the contamination factor to 1/5; B, reducing either snails or exposure to 1/5; and C, reducing the mean longevity of the parasite by treatment to 1/5.

C. The break point. The standard has been modified in A, by reduction of longevity by treatment to 1/5. To this has been added decrease of exposure, or of snails, to give a total reduction of transmission factors to 1/8.75 in B, 1/10 in C, 1/11.25 in D, and 1/15 in E.

D. The rise and fall of a schistosome infection. Happenings after introduction above the break point followed by application of 4 apparently equivalent control programmes in that each reduces one of the factors involved to 1/15 of its original value. (After MacDonald, 1965.)

138

control measures. These were not always what would otherwise have been expected.

MODELS OF *HAEMONCHUS CONTORTUS*

Whereas the models of schistosomes were constructed in order to investigate the factors influencing parasite density and so to plan control measures, the models of the *H. contortus*-sheep system were constructed by Whitlock (1966) and Ratcliffe *et al.* (1969) in order to assist understanding of the natural methods of population regulation of this nematode. The infection cycle of this species has already been considered (pp. 127–128), and there is general agreement that mechanisms exist for regulation of infection levels in individual sheep. These may involve self-cure and regulation around a threshold. The approach adopted by Whitlock and his colleagues was to use the methods of systems analysis, and to concentrate upon the relationships between the parasite population and the flock of sheep. At this level they considered the relationships and the changes in the host-parasite system to be predictable, whereas at the level of the individual sheep and their parasites they were not. Similarly, the major pathological effect of *H. contortus* is anaemia which can be assessed by haematocrit determinations, and whereas the extent of disease suffered by individual animals is variable, some dying whilst others show no physiological disturbance, and relates in part inversely to egg production by the parasite, the extent of disease can be generalised at the level of the parasite population and the host flock.

Threshold values for individual animals were postulated, and a model was constructed of the mechanisms controlling parasite infection levels, showing both the flow of materials and of information (Fig. 34). The sigmoid symbols indicate provision for a function relating two variables, but the exact form of the function must be specified in each case and the variable must exceed a threshold value. The model also takes account of gaps in detailed information, as for example the exact nature of the inhibitor and its mechanism.

Whitlock and his colleagues believed that the parasite biomass was limited in order to avoid drain on the host population, and that the parasite population was constrained to within narrowly predictable limits due to the operation of a number of feedback controls. These homeostatic controls operated to some extent independently of each other and above threshold levels, and their total effect was to influence the rate of egg production by the adult parasites. They operated on different stages of the parasite, and amongst those identified were inhibition of larval moulting, loss of adult worms as a consequence of the host response and overcrowding of the parasite population such that a few specimens per host gave rise to more eggs per female than many per host. In the initial stages of an infection the rate of egg production can be directly related to larval input, but later becomes independent of it as the controls operate. Survival outside the host was not possible in winter, but was achieved by persistent inhibited larvae in sheep. This inhibition was due to one of the feedback controls. This arrangement of homeostatic controls thus permitted survival of the host-parasite system and maintain it in equilibrium. A model for the

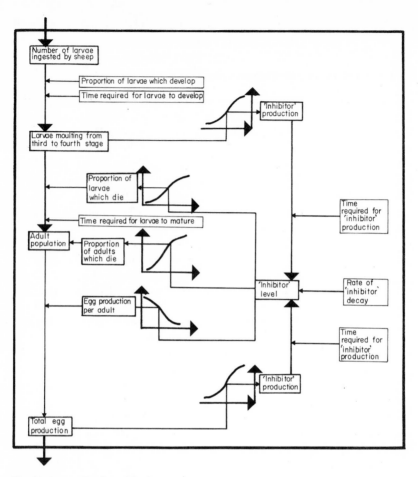

Fig. 34 A postulated model of the parasite control mechanism in the sheep-*Haemonchus contortus* system. Heavy lines represent flows of real quantities, lighter lines flows of information. (After Ratcliffe *et al.*, 1969.)

regulation of haematocrit and its relation to erythrocyte production and egg production was also constructed, and suggestions made as to the ways in which the time variance of the system was controlled (Whitlock *et al.*, 1972) (p. 127).

This model thus summarises concisely the ideas about *Haemonchus* infections and demonstrates the ways in which the parasites can be controlled, as well as giving an indication of the nature and mode and place of action of each control. The authors were also able to provide a reasonable explanation for the life expectancy of any individual sheep, and the model confirms that disease was not the inevitable outcome of infections. They suggested that the maximum capacity of erythrocyte production determined which sheep would die and the relationship between erythrocyte production and erythrocyte deficiency (due to the parasite) determined the degree of anaemia in the sheep that survived. Indeed, they further suggested that it is only the inherently weak sheep that do die. The model has thus greatly assisted understanding of *Haemonchus* population regulation and of haemonchiasis. At the same time it has indicated how valuable methods of systems analysis can be when applied to biological systems and provided the basis for selecting the variables that need to be studied further. It has also served to confirm that parasite populations can be regulated within narrow limits by the operation of a system of negative feedback controls.

GENERAL MODELS OF HOST-PARASITE SYSTEMS

On the basis of his quantitative definition of parasitism, Crofton (1971b) constructed a quantitative model of host-parasite systems such that the essential parameters could be manipulated to give a deeper understanding of the relationship. Due to lack of knowledge of many features such as transmission rates the model is essentially deterministic rather than stochastic.

Crofton assumed that the rate of the host population increase was basically logistic, but that since it never achieved its maximum density due to the lethal effects of the parasite, the actual rate of increase was exponential. He further assumed that parasites were overdispersed throughout their host population in accordance with the negative binomial model, the degree of overdispersion being represented by the parameter k, that there was a lethal level of parasites per host, L, above which the host was killed, and that the reproductive rate of the parasite was higher than that of its host and that this and its potential to infect a host could be represented by an achievement factor, Af. It was not possible to assign values to transmission rates, since it proved impossible to find any quantitative assessment of transmission rates resulting from differences in population size despite the general acceptance that such a relationship exists. It was assumed therefore that transmission rate was directly proportional to the number of hosts.

The model revealed that continued inter-related existence was possible for both host and parasite populations, and the number of both hosts and parasites attained an equilibrium level (Fig. 35A). This could take the form of constant population levels of both, or of constant cyclical changes in host and parasite numbers. When other factors were constant differences in initial infection levels did not affect the equilibrium level but merely the time taken to attain it. Crofton then proceeded to examine the effects of changing values of k, L and Af upon the system. In all cases both populations reached equilibrium level after a time, although the levels differed and there were prolonged and violent oscillations in some cases. The greater the over-dispersion, and so the smaller the value of k, the higher was the equilibrium level. By contrast, as Af increased, the population levels fell and the system became more unstable. The lower the pathogenicity of the parasite (the higher the value of L), the higher the equilibrium level but the greater the instability.

Crofton then went on to consider modifications to this model. The first of these was to consider the effect of sterilisation of heavily infected host individuals. In this case, this was equivalent to death in population terms, and so the same conclusions applied as for changes in L. The second was to consider the

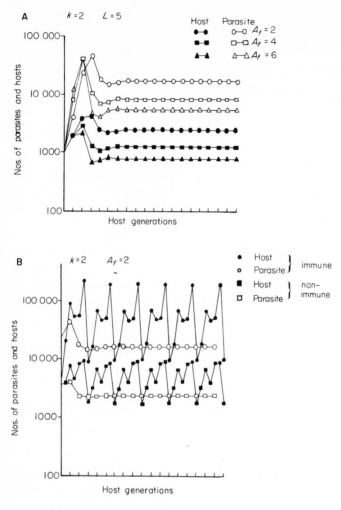

Fig. 35 A computer model of host-parasite relationships. The computed trajectories of host and parasite numbers. (After Crofton, 1971b.)

effect of a host immune response. He assumed that there was a threshold value below which no immunological stimulation took place, and that at the other extreme death could ensue before the response was manifest or effective. He found that in no case did the host and parasite populations now achieve a steady equilibrium level, but that their numbers always oscillated over cycles of generations (Fig. 35B). At high levels of over-dispersion (low k) the oscillations imparted dynamic stability to the systems and maintained the populations at a higher level than in the absence of an immune response. Where k was high the oscillations increased in amplitude, levels overlapped with a non-immune system, and the whole system became increasingly unstable. Thus the model suggests that immune responses produce oscillating systems and that these are more stable when over-dispersion is high. Immune responses, however, do not *necessarily* add stability to systems or invariably result in larger host populations.

The model thus suggests a number of interesting features about host-parasite systems. It confirms that host and parasite populations can persist as a system, with population densities fluctuating around equilibrium levels. Parasites can thus regulate their own population density by the employment of feedback controls, and the host-parasite systems may thus achieve stability. This stability may be dependent upon the ability of parasites to kill their hosts, as verified experimentally by Pennycuick (1971) (p. 85). It was also possible to examine with the model the *population* consequences of immune responses: an aspect that is frequently overlooked. The conclusions were not always what might have been expected; thus an immune response may protect some individuals but not necessarily increase the size of the host population or its stability. The conclusions based on the model must, however, be treated with some caution. It has examined only the special selected features of the host-parasite relationship and their interaction, and has not considered the complexity of other factors that will influence any natural system. These may depress numbers well below the levels considered in the model, and in particular, in many field situations, a lethal level of infection may never be attained at all if parasite numbers are kept low by climatic factors. It is also incorrect to treat L as deterministic, when it is in fact stochastic. Despite this, the model has greatly assisted understanding of the host-parasite relationship by showing how some factors do affect population levels, and the ways in which stability of host-parasite systems may be attained.

MODELS OF *CARYOPHYLLAEUS LATICEPS*

Models of the *C. laticeps*—bream system were constructed by Anderson (1974a, 1974b) in order to describe as succinctly as possible the complex population interaction between host and parasite, and by examining the models for evidence of the attainment of stable equilibria, to achieve some insight into the factors influencing and controlling the dynamics of the host-parasite system. Two approaches towards the description of the life cycle were adopted. The first was deterministic, and attempted eventually to describe the whole life cycle of the parasite, whereas the second was stochastic, and described only the parasite within the fish host.

In the locality from which the field data were obtained, the population changes of *C. laticeps* in bream were very similar to those described earlier in dace (p. 101). The over-dispersion of the parasite throughout the bream population could be described by a negative binomial model. This was not due to the compounding of several waves of random infection but to heterogeneity in the feeding behaviour of the fish, complemented by an over-dispersed distribution of the infected intermediate hosts. The changes in incidence and intensity of infection in bream showed seasonal periodicity in all age groups of the host, although the phase and amplitude of the cycles differed between age classes due to the different feeding habits of the fish. Both host feeding habits and food availability changed seasonally, so that immigration of parasites into the fish was itself a seasonal variable. The survival rate of the parasites in fish decreased in the warmer months, and was not related to population density but was correlated with water temperature and so was also a seasonal variable.

The rate of change of the adult parasite burden in a single fish host could be described in terms of a deterministic model as

$$\frac{dN_t}{dt} = \lambda - \mu N_t$$

where N_t is the number of parasites present at time t and λ and μ are respectively the immigration and death rates. It is assumed that λ is independent of N_t which is true if only the parasites within the fish host are considered, and that μ is independent of parasite density, which has been shown to be the case since it depends on water temperature. The effects of previous infections are ignored.

To produce the seasonal cycles observed, either λ or μ or both must change with time. Field data indicated that both parameters varied with water temperature, and therefore with time, so this condition is fulfilled. Of the three possible equations:

$$\frac{dN_t}{dt} = \lambda(t) - \mu(t)N_t \tag{1}$$

$$\frac{dN_t}{dt} = \lambda - \mu(t)N_t \tag{2}$$

$$\frac{dN_t}{dt} = \lambda(t) - \mu N_t \tag{3}$$

equation (1) is the most appropriate. Thus the combined effects of seasonal immigration and death rates caused the seasonality of parasite changes observed. In this type of equation, unless mortality is exceptionally high, immigration is likely to have the stronger influence on population size.

This deterministic model is over simple, in that it only describes the adult parasites within one host, it ignores the birth process of egg production, the time lags in the system and the chance variation in feeding habits between individual fish. In order to cope with these difficulties Anderson contructed a stochastic model since this could incorporate the variation in transmission rates and the heterogeneous process of the host-parasite interaction, and was better suited to a situation where chance elements are important.

In the stochastic model, immigration rate was assumed to be a random variable, but death rate was correlated with water temperature. Comparison between the observed and expected numbers of C. laticeps immigrants in a single fish was good. The model also predicted a negative binomial distribution of the parasites within the host population, and agreement between this and the observed negative binomial was also good. Finally the comparison between the observed and predicted number of adults per host was also good. Thus the model described the field situation accurately and succinctly. Anderson then proceeded to examine the stability of the host-parasite system in relation to the parameters of immigration and death rates, and natural environmental variables such as water temperature. By using the equivalent stochastic models of equations (1), (2) and (3) above, he showed that when λ is constant, then the temperature dependent death rate has a pronounced effect upon the population, causing severe losses in summer. When μ is constant, the host feeding behaviour has the greatest influence on parasite burden. The combined effects of these parameters cause a peak in numbers in late spring and a depression in summer, as observed in the field. Stability in relation to temperature was examined by simulation, using mean monthly temperature figures over a number of years. In fact, natural variation in water temperature did not markedly affect the stability of the cyclical behaviour of the adult parasite population. The numbers of adults oscillated cyclically, but never reached a steady state due to chance fluctuations around the equilibrium. These occasionally resulted in the adult part of the population becoming extinct, but the population then persisted as larval forms in the intermediate host.

In order to take full account of the interaction between parasites and host populations and all stages in the life cycle, Anderson (1974b) returned to a deterministic approach. With a knowledge of the host population size, the adult parasite population size, the parasite egg production and the distribution of the parasites within the hosts and their lethal level, in the sense of Crofton (1971b), he was able to construct a new model. The parasite numbers then exhibited damped oscillations towards a stable equilibrium, or achieved a stable oscillating equilibrium. The model was very sensitive to changes in immigration and birth rates, and stability was enhanced if the death rate of the host population was related to the number of parasites present in a single host and to the number of hosts, i.e. to the size of the parasite population, its distribution and its lethal level. The model was also sensitive to host population changes since if the final host became too abundant, all the intermediate hosts could be eaten and the parasites become extinct. When the numbers of intermediate hosts were large in relation to the numbers of fish and the levels of infection low, the model led to greater stability in the host-parasite interaction. Stability of $C.$ $laticeps$ was assisted by over-dispersion, since at lethal levels regulation could operate in the manner described by Crofton (1971b), and by the fact that most parasite eggs were produced at a time of minimum population size, so preventing infection of large numbers of intermediate hosts with resulting production of large numbers of larvae.

Thus, despite their limitations, both models did describe the essential features of the $C.$ $laticeps$—bream interaction, and did provide information about the changes in both populations as well as providing insight into the factors controlling and influencing the population levels and their changes.

Appendix

An outline classification of the principal species mentioned in this book with brief notes on their life histories.

Phylum Protozoa
Sub-phylum Sarcomastigophora
Order Kinetoplastida

Trypanosoma lewisi — In blood of rats. Vector the rat flea *Nosopsyllus fasciatus*. Contaminative transmission by ingestion of flea.

T. gambiense (and *T. brucei)* — In blood of humans. Vector tsetse flies, especially *Glossina palpalis*. Inoculative transmission by fly bite.

Leishmania tropica — In blood of humans. Vector the sand fly *Phlebotomus argentipes*. Inoculative transmission by fly bite.

Order Opalinida

Opalina ranarum — One host only. In rectum of frogs.

Sub-phylum Sporozoa
Order Eucoccida

Eimeria tenella (and other *Eimeria* spp.) — Intestine of chickens. Transmission by ingestion of oocysts. One host only.

Plasmodium vivax — Blood of humans. Vector *Anopheles* spp. mosquitoes. Transmission by bite of insect.

P. berghei — Blood of tree rats. Vector as *P. vivax*.

Sub-phylum Ciliophora
Order Hymenostomatida

Ichthyophthirius multifiliis — One host only. On skin of fish.

Phylum Platyhelminthes
Class Monogenea

Entobdella soleae — One host only. Skin of *Solea solea*.
Dactylogyrus vastator — One host only. Gills of *Cyprinus carpio*.
Discocotyle sagittata — One host only. Gills of *Salmo trutta*.

Class Digenea

Fasciola hepatica — Adult in gall bladder of sheep and cattle. Intermediate host *Lymnea truncatula* in Europe, *L. tomentosa* in Australia. Metacercariae encyst on grass.

Diplostomum gasterostei — Adults in intestine of birds. First intermediate host *Lymnea pereger*. Metacercariae in eyes of fish.

Schistosoma mansoni — Adult in blood of human. Intermediate host *Biomphalaria glabrata*. Cercariae penetrate directly. Other species similar.

Class Cestoda
Order Caryophyllidea
Caryophyllaeus laticeps   Adults in intestine of cyprinid fish. Larvae in coelom of aquatic oligochaetes. Transmission by ingestion.

Order Pseudophyllidea
Triaenophorus nodulosus   Adults in intestine of *Esox lucius*, plerocercoid in liver of *Perca fluviatilis*, procercoid in haemocoele of *Cyclops*.

Schistocephalus solidus   Adults in intestine of birds, plerocercoid in body cavity of *Gasterosteus aculeatus*, procercoid in haemocoele of *Cyclops* sp.

Order Proteocephala
Proteocephalus filicollis   Adults in intestine of *Gasterosteus aculeatus*, larva in haemocoele of *Cyclops*.

Order Cyclophyllidea
Hymenolepis diminuta   Adult in intestine of rats. Cysticercoid in haemocoele of *Tribolium confusum* and many other insects. Other species of *Hymenolepis* similar.

Phylum Acanthocephala
Pomphorhynchus laevis   Adults in intestine of cyprinid fish. Larvae in haemocoele of *Gammarus pulex*.

Phylum Aschelminthes
Class Nematoda
Order Ascaroidea
Ascaris lumbricoides   Adults in intestine of pigs. Infection by ingestion of second stage larvae.

Order Filaroidea
Wuchereria bancrofti   Adults in lymph glands of humans. Microfilariae transmitted by *Culex* or *Aedes* mosquitoes.

Onchocerca volvulus   Adults in mesenteries of humans. Microfilariae transmitted by *Simulium damnosum* blackflies.

Order Strongyloidea
Haemonchus contortus   Adult in intestine of sheep. Infection by ingestion of third stage larvae.

Ostertagia ostertagi   Adults in intestine of cattle. Infection by ingestion of third stage larvae.

Nippostrongylus brasiliensis   Adults in intestine of rats. Infection by skin penetration of third stage larvae.

References

ACKERT J.E. (1942) Natural resistance to helminthic infections. *Journal of Parasitology* **28**, 1–14.

ACKERT J.E., GRAHAM G.L., NOLF L.O. and PORTER D.A. (1931) Quantitative studies on the administration of variable numbers of nematode eggs (*Ascaridia lineata*) to chickens. *Transactions of the American Microscopical Society* **50**, 206–214.

ALESANDRO P.A.D. (1970) Nonpathogenic trypanosomes of rodents. In: G.J.Jackson, R.Herman and I.Singer (Ed.). *Immunity to Parasitic Animals.* Vol. 2. pp. 691–738. Appleton-Century-Crofts: New York.

ALLONBY E.W. and URQUHART G.M. (1973) Self-cure of *Haemonchus contortus* infections under field conditons. *Parasitology* **66**, 43–53.

ALPHEY T.J.W. (1970) Studies on the distribution and site location of *Nippostrongylus brasiliensis* within the small intestine of laboratory rats. *Parasitology* **61**, 449–460.

ANDERSON R.M. (1974a) Population dynamics of the cestode *Caryophyllaeus laticeps* (Pallas, 1781) in the bream (*Abramis brama* L.). *Journal of Animal Ecology* **43**, 305–321.

ANDERSON R.M. (1974b) Mathematical models of host-helminth parasite interactions. In: M.B.Usher and M.H.Williamson (Ed.). *Ecological Stability* pp. 43–70. Chapman and Hall: London.

AVERY R.A. (1969) The ecology of tapeworm parasites in wildfowl. *Wildfowl* **20**, 59–68.

AWACHIE J.B.E. (1965) The ecology of *Echinorhynchus truttae* Schrank, 1788 (Acanthocephala) in a trout stream in North Wales. *Parasitology* **55**, 747–762.

AWACHIE J.B.E. (1966) The development and life history of *Echinorhynchus truttae* Schrank, 1788 (Acanthocephala). *Journal of Helminthology* **40**, 11–32.

AWACHIE J.B.E. (1967) Experimental studies on some host-parasite relationships of the Acanthocephala. Co-invasion of *Gammarus pulex* L. by *Echinorhynchus truttae* Schrank, 1788 and *Polymorphus minutus* (Goeze, 1782). *Acta Parasitologica Polonica* **15**, 69–74.

BAER J.G. (Ed.) (1957) *First Symposium on Host Specificity among Parasites of Vertebrates.* Paul Attinger: Neuchâtel.

BAILEY G.N.A. (1971) *Hymenolepis diminuta*: circadian rhythm in movement and body length in the rat. *Experimental Parasitology* **29**, 285–291.

BAKKE T.A. (1972) Studies on the helminth fauna of Norway XXII: The common gull, *Larus canus* L., as final host for Digenea (Platyhelminthes). 1. The ecology of the common gull and the infection in relation to the season and the gull's habitat, together with the distribution of the parasites in the intestine. *Norwegian Journal of Zoology* **20**, 165–188.

BAUER O.N. (1962) The ecology of parasites of freshwater fish. In: *Parasites of freshwater fish and the biological basis for their control.* I.P.S.T.: Jerusalem.

BERRIE A.D. (1970) Snail problems in African Schistosomiasis. *Advances in Parasitology* **8**, 43–96.

BORAY J.C. (1966) Studies on the relative susceptibility of some lymnaeids to infection with *Fasciola hepatica* and *F. gigantica* and on the adaptation of *Fasciola* spp. *Annals of Tropical Medicine and Parasitology* **60**, 114–124.

BORAY J.C. (1969) Experimental fascioliasis in Australia. *Advances in Parasitology* **7**, 96–210.

BRADLEY D.J. (1974) Stability in host-parasite systems. In: M.B.Usher and M.H.Williamson (Ed.). *Ecological Stability.* pp. 71–88. Chapman and Hall: London.

BROOKS W.M. (1969) Molluscan Immunity to Metazoan Parasites. In: G.J.Jackson, R.Herman and I.Singer (Ed.). *Immunity to Parasitic Animals.* Vol. 1. pp. 149–171. Appleton-Century-Crofts: New York.

BRATEN T. and HOPKINS C.A. (1969) The migration of *Hymenolepis diminuta* in the rat's intestine during normal development and following surgical implantation. *Parasitology* **59**, 891–905.

BULL P.C. (1964) Ecology of helminth parasites of the wild rabbit *Oryctolagus cuniculus* in New Zealand. *Bulletin of the New Zealand Department of Scientific and Industrial Research* **158**, 1–147.

CABLE R.M. (1972) Behaviour of digenetic trematodes. In: E.U.Canning and C.A.Wright (Ed.). *Behavioural Aspects of Parasite Transmission. Zoological Journal of the Linnean Society* **51**, Suppl. 1, 1–18.

CHAPPELL L.H. (1969) The parasites of the three-spined stickleback *Gasterosteus aculeatus* L. from a Yorkshire pond. 1. Seasonal variation of parasite fauna. *Journal of Fish Biology* **1**, 137–152.

CHENG T.C. (1971) Enhanced growth as a manifestation of parasitism and shell deposition in parasitised molluscs. In: T.C.Cheng (Ed.). *Aspects of the Biology of Symbiosis*. pp. 103–136. University Park Press: Baltimore.

CHERNIN E. (1952) The relapse phenomenon in the *Leucocytozoon simondi* infection of the domestic duck. *American Journal of Hygiene* **56**, 101–118.

CHUBB J.C. (1963a) On the characterisation of the parasite fauna of the fish of Llyn Tegid. *Proceedings of the Zoological Society of London,* **141**, 609–621.

CHUBB J.C. (1963b) Seasonal occurrence and maturation of *Triaenophorus nodulosus* (Pallas, 1781) (Cestoda: Pseudophyllidea) in the pike *Esox lucius* L. of Llyn Tegid. *Parasitology* **53**, 419–433.

CHUBB J.C. (1964) Observations on the occurrence of the plerocercoids of *Triaenophorus nodulosus* (Pallas, 1781) (Cestoda: Pseudophyllidea) in the perch *Perca fluviatilis* L. of Llyn Tegid (Bala Lake) Merioneth. *Parasitology* **54**, 481–491.

CHUBB J.C. (1967) A review of seasonal occurrence and maturation of tapeworms in British freshwater fish. *Parasitology* **53**, 13P.

CIORDIA H. and BIZZELL W.E. (1963) The effects of various constant temperatures on the development of the free living stages of some nematode parasites of cattle. *Journal of Parasitology* **49**, 60–63.

COLE L.C. (1954) The population consequences of life history phenomena. *Quarterly Review of Biology* **29**, 103–137.

CROFTON H.D. (1963) Nematode parasite populations in sheep and on pasture. *Commonwealth Agricultural Bureau Publications* No. 35, 1–104.

CROFTON H.D. (1966) *Nematodes*. Hutchinson and Co.: London.

CROFTON H.D. (1971a) A quantitative approach to parasitism. *Parasitology* **62**, 179–193.

CROFTON H.D. (1971b) A model of host-parasite relationships. *Parasitology* **63**, 343–364.

CROLL N.A. (1972) Behaviour of larval nematodes. In: E.U.Canning and C.A.Wright (Ed.). *Behavioural aspects of Parasite Transmission. Zoological Journal of the Linnean Society,* Suppl. **1**, 31–52.

CROMPTON D.W.T. (1970) *An Ecological Approach to Acanthocephalan Physiology*. University Press: Cambridge.

CROMPTON D.W.T. (1973) The sites occupied by some parasitic helminths in the alimentary tract of vertebrates. *Biological Reviews* **48**, 27–83.

CUCKLER A.C. (1970) Coccidiosis and Histomoniasis in Avian Hosts. In: G.J.Jackson, R.Herman and J.Singer (Ed.). *Immunity to Parasitic Animals*. Vol. 2. pp. 371–397. Appleton-Century-Crofts: New York.

DAWES B. and HUGHES D.L. (1964) Fascioliasis: the invasive stages of *Fasciola hepatica* in mammalian hosts. *Advances in Parasitology* **2**, 97–168.

DAMIAN R.T. (1964) Molecular mimicry: antigen sharing by parasite and host and its consequences. *American Naturalist* **98**, 129–149.

DESOWITZ R.S. (1963) Adaptations of trypanosomes to abnormal hosts. *Annals of the New York Academy of Sciences* **113**, 74–87.

DESOWITZ R.S. (1970) African Trypanosomes. In: G.J.Jackson, R.Herman and J.Singer (Ed.). *Immunity to Parasitic Animals*. Vol. 2. pp. 551–596. Appleton-Century-Crofts: New York.

DINEEN J.K. (1963) Immunological aspects of parasitism. *Nature, London* **197**, 268–269.

DINEEN J.K., DONALD A.D., WAGLAND B.M. and OFFNER J. (1965) The dynamics of the host-parasite relationship III. The response of sheep to primary infections with *Haemonchus contortus*. *Parasitology* **55**, 515–525.

DIXON K.E. (1966) The physiology of excystment of the metacercaria of *Fasciola hepatica* L. *Parasitology* **56**, 431–456.

DOGIEL V.A. (1961) Ecology of the parasites of freshwater fishes. In: V.A.Dogiel, G.K.Petrushevski and Yu.I.Polyanski (Ed.). *Parasitology of Fishes*. pp. 1–47. Oliver and Boyd: Edinburgh and London.

DOGIEL V.A. (1964) *General Parasitology*. Oliver and Boyd: Edinburgh and London.

DONALD A.D., DINEEN J.K. and ADAMS D.B. (1969) The dynamics of the host-parasite relationship VII. The effect of discontinuity of infection on resistance to *Haemonchus contortus* in sheep. *Parasitology* **59**, 497–503.

DUKE B.O.L. (1971) The ecology of onchocerciasis in man and animals. In: A.M.Fallis (Ed.). *Ecology and Physiology of Parasites*. pp. 213–222. Adam Hilger Ltd.: London.

DUKE B.O.L. (1972) Behavioural aspects of the life cycle of *Loa*. In: E.U.Canning and C.A.Wright (Ed.). *Behaviorual aspects of Parasite Transmission. Zoological Journal of the Linnean Society* **51**, Suppl. **1**, 97–107.

DUKE B.O.L. and WIJERS D.J.B. (1958) Studies on loiasis in monkeys: the relationship between human and simian *Loa* in the rain forest zone of the British Cameroons. *Annals of Tropical Medicine and Parasitology* **52**, 158–175.

DUXBURY R.E., MOON A.P. and SADUN E.H. (1961) Susceptibility and resistance of *Anopheles quadrimaculatus* to *Dirofilaria uniformis. Journal of Parasitology* **47**, 687–692.

EL MOFTY M.M. and SMYTH J.D. (1959) Endocrine control of sexual reproduction in *Opalina ranarum* parasitic in *Rana temporaria. Nature, London* **186**, 559.

ERASMUS D.A. (1959) The migration of *Cercaria X* Baylis (Strigeida) within the fish intermediate host. *Parasitology* **49**, 173–190.

ESCH G.W. (1971) Impact of ecological succession on the parasite fauna in centrachids from oligotrophic and eutrophic ecosystems. *American Midland Naturalist* **86**, 160–168.

FERGUSON M.S. (1943) Migration and localisation of an animal parasite within the host. *Journal of Experimental Zoology* **93**, 375–403.

FISCHER H. (1967) The life cycle of *Proteocephalus fluviatilis* Bangham (Cestoda) from smallmouth bass, *Micropterus dolomieui* Lacepede. *Canadian Journal of Zoology* **46**, 569–579.

FISCHER H. and FREEMAN R.S. (1969) Penetration of parenteral plerocercoids of *Proteocephalus ambloplitis* (Leidy) into the gut of smallmouth bass. *Journal of Parasitology* **55**, 766–774.

GARNHAM P.C.C. (1964) Factors influencing the development of protozoa in their arthropodoan hosts. *Symposia of the British Society for Parasitology* **2**, 33–50.

GARNHAM P.C.C. (1970) Primate Malaria. In: G.J.Jackson, R.Herman and J.Singer (Ed.). *Immunity to Parasitic Animals* Vol. 2. pp. 767–791. Appleton-Century-Crofts: New York.

GATEHOUSE A.G. (1972) Host finding behaviour of tsetse flies. In: E.U.Canning and C.A.Wright (Ed.). *Behavioural aspects of Parasite transmission. Zoological Journal of the Linnean Society* **51**, Suppl. **1**, 83–95.

GILLIES M.T. (1972) Some aspects of mosquito behaviour in relation to the transmission of parasites In: E.U.Canning and C.A.Wright (Ed.). *Behavioural aspects of Parasite transmission. Zoological Journal of the Linnean Society* **51**, Suppl. **1**, 69–81.

GOBLE F.C. (1970) South American Trypanosomes. In: G.J.Jackson, R.Herman and J.Singer (Ed.). *Immunity to Parasite Animals.* Vol. 2. pp. 597–689. Appleton-Century-Crofts: New York.

GOODALL I. (1972) The growth of *Hymenolepis microstoma* in the laboratory rat. *Parasitology* **65**, 137–142.

GRAY J.S. (1972a) The effect of host age on the course of infection of *Raillietina cesticillus* (Molin, 1858) in the fowl. *Parasitology* **65**, 235–241.

GRAY J.S. (1972b) Studies on the course of infection of the poultry cestode *Raillietina cesticillus* (Molin, 1858) in the definitive host. *Parasitology* **65**, 243–250.

GRAY J.S. (1973) Studies on host resistance to secondary infections of *Raillietina cesticillus* (Molin, 1858) in the fowl. *Parasitology* **67**, 375–382.

HAIRSTON N.G. (1965) On the mathematical analysis of schistosome populations. *Bulletin of the World Health Organisation* **33**, 45–62.

HALVORSEN O. and ANDERSEN K. (1974) Some effects of population density in infections with *Diphyllobothrium dendriticum* (Nitzsch) in golden hamster (*Mesocricetus auratus* Waterhouse) and common gull (*Larus canus* L.). *Parasitology* **69**, 149–160.

HALVORSEN O. and WISSLER K. Studies on the helminth fauna of Norway, XXVIII: An experimental study of the ability of *Diphyllobothrium latum* (L.), *D. dendriticum* (Nitzsch) and *D. ditremum* (Creplin) (Cestoda: Pseudophyllidea) to infect paratenic hosts. *Norwegian Journal of Zoology* **21**, 201–210.

HALVORSEN O. and WILLIAMS H.H. (1968) Studies of the helminth fauna of Norway IX: *Gyrocotyle*

(Platyhelminthes) in *Chimaera monstrosa* from Oslo Fjord, with emphasis on its mode of attachment and a regulation in the degree of infection. *Nytt Magasin for Zoologi* 15, 130–142.

HAMMOND D.M. (1971) The development and ecology of coccidia and related intracellular parasites. In: A.M.Fallis (Ed.). *Ecology and physiology of parasites.* pp. 3–20. Adam Hilger Ltd.: London.

HAWKING F. (1968) The 24-hour periodicity of microfilariae: bilogical mechanisms responsible for its production and control *Proceedings of the Royal Society,* B, 169, 59–76.

HINE P.M. and KENNEDY C.R. (1974a) Observations on the distribution specificity and pathogenicity of the acanthocephalan *Pomphorhynchus laevis* (Muller). *Journal of Fish Biology* 6, 521–535.

HINE P.M. and KENNEDY C.R. (1974b) The population biology of the acanthocephalan *Pomphorhynchus laevis* (Muller) in the River Avon. *Journal of Fish Biology* 6, 665–679.

HOLMES J.C. (1961) Effects of concurrent infections on *Hymenolepis diminuta* (Cestoda) and *Moniliformis dubius* (Acanthocephala). 1. General effects and comparison with crowding. *Journal of Parasitology* 47, 209–216.

HOLMES J.C. and BETHEL W.M. (1972) Modification of intermediate host behaviour by parasites. In: E.U.Canning and C.A.Wright (Ed.) *Behavioural aspects of Parasite transmission. Journal of the Linnean Society* 51, Suppl. 1, 123–149.

HOPKINS C.A. (1959) Seasonal variations in the incidence and development of the cestode *Proteocephalus filicollis* (Rud. 1810) in *Gasterosteus aculeatus* (L. 1766). *Parasitology* 49, 529–542.

HOPKINS C.A. (1970) Diurnal movement of *Hymenolepis diminuta* in the rat. *Parasitology* 60, 225–271.

HOPKINS C.A., SUBRAMANIAN G. and STALLARD H. (1972) The development of *Hymenolepis diminuta* in primary and secondary infections in mice. *Parasitology* 64, 401–412.

HORAK I.G. (1971) Paramphistomiasis of domestic ruminants. *Advances in Parasitology* 9, 33–72.

HORTON-SMITH C. and LONG P.L. (1963) Coccidia and coccidiosis in the domestic fowl and turkey. *Advances in Parasitology* 1, 68–107.

HUFF C.G. (1929) The effects of selection upon susceptibility to bird malaria in *Culex pipiens* Linn. *Annals of Tropical Medicine and Parasitology* 23, 427–438.

HYNES H.B.N. and NICHOLAS W.L. (1963) The importance of the acanthocephalan *Polymorphus minutus* as a parasite of the domestic ducks in the United Kingdom. *Journal of Helminthology* 37, 185–198.

IKEME M.M. (1971) Effects of different levels of nutrition and continuing dosing of poultry with *Ascaridia galli* eggs on the subsequent development of parasite populations. *Parasitology* 63, 233–250.

JAMES B.L. (1965) The effects of parasitism by larval Digenea on the digestive gland of the intertidal prosobranch, *Littorina saxatilis* (Olivi) subsp. *tenebrosa* (Montagu). *Parasitology* 55, 93–115.

JAMES B.L. (1968a) The occurrence of *Parvatrema homoeotecnum* James, 1964 (Trematoda: Gymnophallidae) in a population of *Littorina saxatilis tenebrosa* (Mont.). *Journal of Natural History* 2, 21–37.

JAMES B.L. (1968b) The occurrence of larval Digenea in ten species of intertidal prosobranch molluscs in Cardigan Bay. *Journal of Natural History* 2, 329–343.

JAMES B.L. (1971) Host selection and ecology of marine digenean larvae. In: D.J.Crisp (Ed.). *Fourth European Marine Biology Symposium:* pp. 179–196. University Press: Cambridge.

JARRETT E.E.E., JARRETT W.F.H. and URQUHART G.M. (1968) Quantitative studies on the kinetics of establishment and expulsion of intestinal nematodes in susceptible and immune hosts. *Nippostrongylus brasiliensis* in the rat. *Parasitology* 58, 625–639.

JOYNER L.P. (1969) Immunological variation between two strains of *Eimeria acervulina. Parasitology* 59, 725–732.

JOYNER L.P. and NORTON C.C. (1973) The immunity arising from continuous low-level infection with *Eimeria tenella. Parasitology* 67, 333–340.

KEARN G.C. (1966) The life cycle of the monogenean *Entobdella soleae,* a skin parasite of the common sole. *Parasitology* 53, 253–263.

KEARN G.C. (1967) Experiments on host finding and host-specificity in the monogenean skin parasite *Entobdella soleae. Parasitology* 57, 585–605.

KEARN G.C. (1973) An endogenous circadian hatching rhythm in the monogenean skin parasite *Entobdella soleae,* and its relationship to the activity rhythm of the host (*Solea solea*). *Parasitology* 66, 101–122.

151

KEARN G.C. (1974) The effects of skin fish mucus on hatching in the monogenean parasite *Entobdella soleae* from the skin of the common sole, *Solea solea*. *Parasitology* **68**, 173–188.

KENNEDY C.R. (1969a) The occurrence of *Eubothrium crassum* (Cestoda: Pseudophyllidea) in salmon *Salmo salar* and trout, *S. trutta*, of the River Exe. *Journal of Zoology* **157**, 1–9.

KENNEDY C.R. (1969b) Seasonal incidence and development of the cestode *Caryophyllaeus laticeps* (Pallas) in the River Avon. *Parasitology* **59**, 783–794.

KENNEDY C.R. (1971) The effect of temperature upon the establishment and survival of the cestode *Caryophyllaeus laticeps* in orfe, *Leuciscus idus*. *Parasitology* **63**, 59–66.

KENNEDY C.R. (1972) The effect of the cestode *Caryophyllaeus laticeps* upon production and respiration of its intermediate host. *Parasitology* **64**, 485–499.

KENNEDY C.R. (1974) The importance of parasite mortality in regulating the population size of the acanthocephalan *Pomphorhynchus laevis* in goldfish. *Parasitology* **68**, 93–101.

KUNTZ R.E. (1952) *Schistosoma mansoni* and *S. haematobium* in the Yemen, S.W. Arabia; with a report on an unusual factor in the epidemiology of schistosomiasis *mansoni*. *Journal of Parasitology* **38**, 24–28.

LAINSON R. and SHAW J.J. (1971) Epidemiological considerations of the leishmanias with particular reference to the New World. In: A.M.Fallis (Ed.). *Ecology and Physiology of Parasites*. pp. 21–56. Adam Hilger Ltd.: London.

LESTER R.J.G. (1972) Attachment of *Gyrodactylus* to *Gasterosteus* and host response. *Journal of Parasitology* **58**, 717–722.

LESTER R.J.G. and ADAMS J.R. (1974) A simple model of a *Gyrodactylus* population. *International Journal of Parasitology* **4**, 497–506.

LEWERT R.M. (1970 Schistosomes. In: G.J.Jackson, R.Herman and I.Singer (Ed.). *Immunity to parasitic animals*. Vol. 2. pp. 981–1008. Appleton-Century-Crofts: New York.

LEWERT R.M. and MANDLOWITZ S. (1963) Innate immunity to *Schistosoma mansoni* relative to the state of the connective tissue. In: T.C.Cheng (Ed.). *Some biochemical and immunological aspects of host-parasite relationships*. Annals of the New York Academy of Sciences **113**, 54–62.

LIE K.Y., BASCH P.F. and UMATHERY T. (1965) Antagonism between two species of larval trematodes in the same snail. *Nature, London* **206**, 422–423.

LLEWELLYN J. (1956) The host-specificity, micro-ecology, adhesive attitudes, and comparative morphology of some trematode gill parasites. *Journal of the marine Biology Association of the United Kingdom* **35**, 113–127.

LLEWELLYN J. (1957) Specificity of Monogenea. In: J.G.Baer (Ed.). *First Symposium on Host Specificity among Parasites of Vertebrates*. Paul Attinger: Neuchâtel.

LONG P.L. (1967) Studies on *Eimeria praecox* Johnson, 1930, in the chicken. *Parasitology* **57**, 351–361.

LUND E.E. (1967) Acquired resistance to experimental *Heterakis* infections in chickens and turkeys; effect on the transmission of *Histomonas meleagrides*. *Journal of Helminthology* **41**, 55–62.

MCCAIG M.L.O. and HOPKINS C.A. (1963) Studies on *Schistocephalus solidus*. II. Establishment and longevity in the definitive host. *Experimental Parasitology* **13**, 273–283.

MACDONALD G. (1957) *The Epidemiology and Control of Malaria*. Oxford University Press: London.

MACDONALD G. (1965) The dynamics of helminth infections with special reference to schistosomes. *Transactions of the Royal Society of Tropical Medicine and Hygiene* **59**, 489–506.

MCGHEE R.B. (1970) Avian Malaria. In: G.J.Jackson, R.Herman and J.Singer (Ed.). *Immunity to Parasitic Animals* Vol. 2. pp. 331–369. Appleton-Century-Crofts: New York.

MACINNIS A.J. (1965) Responses of *Schistosoma mansoni* miracidia to chemical attractants. *Journal of Parasitology* **51**, 731–746.

MACKENZIE K. and GIBSON D. (1970) Ecological studies on some parasites of plaice, *Pleuronectes platessa* (L) and flounder, *Platichthys flesus* (L.). *Symposia of the British Society for Parasitology* **8**, 1–42.

MCVICAR A.H. and FLETCHER T.C. (1970) Serum factors in *Raja radiata* toxic to *Acanthobothrium quadripartitum* (Cestoda: Tetraphyllidea), a parasite specific to *R. naevus*. *Parasitology* **61**, 55–63.

MICHAELOW V. (1955) On some problems of the inter-relations between first intermediate hosts and the cestode larvae. *Zoologichesko Zhurnal* **34**, 986–991.

MICHEL J.F. (1969) The epidemiology and control of some nematode infections of grazing animals. *Advances in Parasitology* **7**, 211–282.

MICHEL J.F. (1970) The regulation of populations of *Ostertagia ostertagi* in calves. *Parasitology* **61**, 435–447.

152

MILSUM J.H. (1967) *Biological Control System Analysis.* McGraw-Hill: New York.

MOSS G.D. (1971) The nature of the immune response of the mouse to the bile duct cestode *Hymenolepis microstoma. Parasitology* **62,** 285–294.

MUELLER J.F. (1968) Growth stimulating effect of experimental sparganosis in thyroidectomised and hypophysectomised rats, and comparative activity of different species of *Spirometra. Journal of Parasitology* **54,** 795–801.

NELSON G.S. (1964) Factors influencing the development and behaviour of filarial nematodes in their arthropodan hosts. *Symposia of the British Society for Parasitology* **2,** 75–119.

NELSON G.S. (1970) Onchocerciasis. *Advances in Parasitology* **8,** 173–224.

NELSON G.S. (1972) Human behaviour in the transmission of parasitic diseases. In: E.U.Canning and C.A.Wright (Ed.). *Behavioural Aspects of Parasite Transmission. Zoological Journal of the Linnean Society* **51,** Suppl. **1,** 109–122.

NIGRELLI R.F. (1935) On the effect of fish mucus on *Epibdella melleni,* a monogenetic trematode of marine fishes. *Journal of Parasitology* **21,** 6–15.

NIGRELLI R.F. (1937) Further studies on the susceptibility and acquired immunity of marine fishes to *Epibdella melleni,* a monogenetic trematode. *Zoologica, New York* **22,** 185–197.

OGILVIE B.M. and JONES V.E. (1971) *Nippostrongylus brasiliensis:* a review of immunity and the host-parasite relationship in the rat. *Experimental Parasitology* **29,** 138–177.

ORR T.S.C., HOPKINS C.A. and CHARLES G.H. (1969) Host specificity and rejection of *Schistocephalus solidus. Parasitology* **59,** 683–690.

PALING J.E. (1965) The population dynamics of the monogenean gill parasite *Discocotyle sagittata* Leuckart on Windermere trout, *Salmo truta* L. *Parasitology* **55,** 667–694.

PENNYCUICK L. (1971) Frequency distributions of parasites in a population of three-spined sticklebacks, *Gasterosteus aculeatus* L., with particular reference to the negative binomial distribution. *Parasitology* **63,** 389–406.

RADKE M.G., RITCHIE L.S. and ROWAN W.B. (1961) Effects of water velocities on worm burdens of animals exposed to *Schistosoma mansoni* cercariae released under laboratory and field conditions. *Experimental Parasitology* **11,** 323–331.

RATCLIFFE L.H., TAYLOR H.M., WHITLOCK J.H. and LYNN W.R. (1969) Systems analysis of a host-parasite interaction. *Parasitology* **59,** 649–661.

ROBERTS L.S. (1961) The influence of population density on patterns and physiology of growth in *Hymenolepis diminuta* (Cestoda: Cyclophyllidea) in the definitive host. *Experimental Parasitology* **11,** 332–371.

ROBERTS L.S. (1966) Developmental physiology of cestodes I. Host dietary carbohydrate and the crowding effect in *Hymenolepis diminuta. Experimental Parasitology* **18,** 305–310.

ROGERS W.P. (1962) *The Nature of Parasitism.* Academic Press: London and New York.

ROGERS W.P. and SOMMERVILLE R.I. (1963) The infective stage of nematode parasites and its significance in parasitism. *Advances in Parasitology* **1,** 109–177.

ROSE M.E. (1967) Immunity to *Eimeria brunetti* and *Eimeria maxima* infections in the fowl. *Parasitology* **57,** 363–370.

ROTHMAN A.H. (1959) Studies on the excystment of tapeworms. *Experimental Parasitology* **8,** 336–364.

ROTHSCHILD M. and FORD B. (1964) Breeding of the rabbit flea (*Spilopsyllus cuniculi*) (Dale) controlled by the reproductive hormones of the host. *Nature, London* **201,** 103.

ROWAN W.B. (1956) The mode of hatching of the egg of *Fasciola hepatica. Experimental Parasitology* **5,** 118–137.

SCHAD G.A. (1963) Niche diversification in a parasite species flock. *Nature, London* **198,** 404–406.

SCHAD G.A. (1966) Immunity, competition and natural regulation of helminth populations. *American Naturalist* **100,** 359–364.

SMITHERS S.R. (1968) Immunity to blood helminths. *Symposia of the British Society for Parasitology* **6,** 55–66.

SMITHERS S.R. and TERRY R.J. (1969) The immunology of schistosomiasis. *Advances in Parasitology* **7,** 41–93.

SMYTH J.D. (1952) Studies on tapeworm physiology VI. Effect of temperature on the maturation *in vitro* of *Schistocephalus solidus. Journal of Experimental Biology* **29,** 304–309.

SMYTH J.D. (1962) *Introduction to Animal Parasitology.* English Universities Press Ltd.: London.

SMYTH J.D. (1969) Parasites as biological models. *Parasitology* **59,** 73–91.

SPRENT J.F.A. (1962) Parasitism, immunity and evolution. In: G.W.Leeper (Ed.). *The Evolution of Living Organsims*. pp. 149–165. Melbourne University Press: Melbourne.

SPRENT J.F.A. (1969) Evolutionary aspects of immunity in zooparasitic infections. In: G.J.Jackson, R.Herman and I.Singer (Ed.). *Immunity to Parasitic Animals* Vol. 1. pp. 3–62. Appleton-Century-Crofts: New York.

STIREWELT M.A. (1963) Seminar on immunity to parasitic helminths IV. Schistosome infections. *Experimental Parasitology* **13**, 18–44.

STIREWELT M.A. (1971) Penetration stimuli for schistosome cercariae. In: T.C.Cheng (Ed.) *Aspects of the Biology of Symbiosis*. University Park Press: Baltimore.

STAUBER L.A. (1970) Leishmaniasis. In: G.J.Jackson, R.Herman and I.Singer (Ed.). *Immunity to Parasitic Animals* Vol. 2. pp. 739–765. Appleton-Century-Crofts: New York.

STOHLER H. (1957 Analyse des infectionsverlaufes von *Plasmodium gallinaceum* in darme von *Aedes aegypti*. *Acta Tropica* **14**, 303–326.

TALIAFERRO W.H. (1932) Trypanocidal and reproduction-inhibiting antibodies to *Trypanosoma lewisi* in rats and rabbits. *American Journal of Hygiene* **16**, 32–84.

TERZIAN L.A., STAHLER N. and IRREVERRE F. (1956) The effects of ageing, and the modifications of these effects, on the immunity of mosquitoes to malarial infection. *Journal of Immunology* **76**, 308–318.

THREFALL W. (1967) Studies on the helminth parasites of the herring gull, *Larus argentatus* Pontopp., in North Caernarvonshire and Anglesey. *Parasitology* **57**, 431–453.

THOMAS J.D. (1964) A comparison between the helminth burdens of male and female brown trout, *Salmo trutta* L., from a natural population in the River Teify, West Wales. *Parasitology* **54**, 263–272.

THOMAS J.D. (1965) Studies on some aspects of the ecology of *Mesocoelium monodi*, a trematode parasite of reptiles and amphibia. *Proceedings of the Zoological Society of London* **145**, 471–494.

TRIPP M.R. (1969) General principles and mechanisms of invertebrate immunity. In: G.J.Jackson, R.Herman and I.Singer (Ed.). *Immunity to Parasitic Animals* Vol. 1. pp. 111–128. Appleton-Century-Crofts: New York.

TURNER J.H., KATES K.C. and WILSON G.I. (1962) The interaction of concurrent infections of the abomasal nematodes *Haemonchus contortus*, *Ostertagia circumcincta* and *Trichostrongylus axei* (Trichostrongylidae) in lambs. *Proceedings of the Helminthological Society of Washington* **29**, 210–216.

ULMER M.J. (1971) Site-finding behaviour in helminths in intermediate and definitive hosts. In: A.M.Fallis (Ed.) *Ecology and Physiology of Parasites*. pp. 123–159. Adam Hilger Ltd.: London.

VICKERMAN K. (1971) Morphological and Physiological considerations of extracellular blood Protozoa. In: A.M.Fallis (Ed.). *Ecology and Physiology of Parasites* pp. 58–89. Adam Hilger Ltd.: London.

VOGE M. and BERNTZEN A.K. (1961) *In vitro* hatching of oncospheres of *Hymenolepis diminuta* (Cestoda: Cyclophyllidea). *Journal of Parasitology* **47**, 813–818.

WAGLAND B.M. and DINEEN J.K. (1967) The dynamics of the host-parasite relationship. VI Regeneration of the immune response in sheep infected with *Haemonchus contortus*. *Parasitology* **57**, 59–65.

WALKEY M. and MEAKINS R.H. (1970) An attempt to balance the energy budget of a host-parasite system. *Journal of Fish Biology* **2**, 361–372.

WEINMANN C.J. (1966) Immunity mechanisms in cestode infections. In: E.J.L.Soulsby (Ed.). *Biology of Parasites*. pp. 301–320. Academic Press: New York.

WEINMANN C.J. (1970) Cestodes and Acanthocephala. In: G.J.Jackson, R.Herman and I.Singer (Ed.). *Immunity to Parasitic Animals*. Vol. 2. pp. 1021–1059. Appleton-Century-Crofts: New York.

WHITLOCK J.H. (1966) The environmental biology of a nematode. In: E.J.L.Soulsby (Ed.). *Biology of Parasites* pp. 185–197. Academic Press: New York.

WHITLOCK J.H., CROFTON H.D. and GEORGI J.R. (1972) Characteristics of parasite populations in endemic trichostrongylidosis. *Parasitology* **64**, 413–427.

WILLIAMS R.B. (1973) Effects of different infection rates on the oocyst production of *Eimeria acervulina* or *Eimeria tenella* in the chicken. *Parasitology* **67**, 279–288.

WILLIAMS H.H. (1960) The intestine in members of the genus *Raja* and host-specificity in the Tetraphyllidea. *Nature, London* **188**, 514–516.

154

WILSON R.A. (1967) The structure and permeability of the shell and vitelline membrane of the egg of *Fasciola hepatica. Parasitology* **57**, 47–58.

WILSON R.A. (1968) The hatching mechanism of the egg of *Fasciola hepatica. Parasitology* **58**, 78–89.

WILSON R.A. and DENISON J. (1970) Short-chain fatty acids as stimulants of turning activity by the miracidium of *Fasciola hepatica. Comparative Biochemistry and Physiology* **32**, 511–517.

WILSON E.O. and BOSSERT W.H. (1971) *A Primer of Population Biology.* Sinauer Associates, Inc.: Connecticut.

WISNIEWSKI W.L. (1958) Characterisation of the parasite fauna of an eutrophic lake (Parasitofauna of the biocoenosis of Druzno Lake—Part 1). *Acta Parasitica Polonica* **6**, 1–64.

WISNIEWSKI W.L., SZYMANIK K. and BAZANSKA K. (1958) The formation of a structure in tapeworm populations. *Ceskoslovakia Parasitologia* **5**, 195–212.

WORMS M.J. (1972) Circadian and seasonal rhythms in blood parasites. In: E.U.Canning, C.A.Wright (Ed.). *Behavioural Aspects of Parasite Transmission. Zoological Journal of the Linnean Society* **51**, Suppl. 1, 53–67.

WRIGHT C.A. (1959) Host-location by trematode miracidia. *Annals of Tropical Medicine and Parasitology* **53**, 288–292.

WRIGHT C.A. (1964) Biochemical variation in *Lymnea peregra* (Mollusca, Basommatophora). *Proceedings of the Zoological Society of London* **142**, 371–378.

WRIGHT C.A. (1966a) Miracidial responses to molluscan stimuli. *Proceedings of the First International Congress of Parasitology (Rome, 1964)*, 1058.

WRIGHT C.A. (1966b) The pathogenesis of helminths in the mollusca. *Helminthological abstracts* **35**, 207–224.

WRIGHT C.A. (1970) The ecology of African schistosomiasis. In: G.P.Garlick and R.W.I.Keay (Ed.). *Human Ecology in the Tropics.* pp. 67–80. Pergamon Press: London.

WRIGHT C.A. (1971) *Flukes and Snails.* George Allen and Unwin Ltd.: London.

ZUCKERMAN A. (1970) Malaria of lower mammals. In: G.J.Jackson, R.Herman and I.Singer (Ed.). *Immunity to Parasitic Animals.* Vol. 2. pp. 793–829. Appleton-Century-Crofts: New York.

Index

Bold type indicates an illustration

Overcrowding
    dangers of, 2, 5, 7
    prevention of, 3–5, 7
Overdispersion
    definition, 1
    examples of, 67, **68**, 69, 85–86
    population regulation, 5, 6, 56, 85–87,
        141–143
Oxygen, 50, 72, 73

Paramphistomum microbothrium
    specificity, 32
Parasitism
    nature of, 1
    evolution of, 6, 26–27
Paratenic hosts, 15
Parvatrema homoeotecnum
    dispersion of, 69, **70**, 71
    effects on host, 81
    seasonal changes, 81
Penetration of hosts, 19, 34, 36, 37, 76–77, 79
Periodicity of behaviour, 22, 34, 49–51
Peritrophic membrane, 37, 76–78
pH, 17
Phagocytosis, 27, 34, 38, 84, 115, 118
Phyllodistomum folium
    other species, 57
Phylogenetic aspects of specificity, 27–28, 29
Plasmodium berghei
    course of infection, 118
    cross immunity, 59
    life cycle, 146
Plasmodium cathemerium
    vector resistance to, 34, 77
Plasmodium chabaudi
    population changes, 118
Plasmodium falciparum
    immunity to, 118
Plasmodium gallinaceum
    penetration of vector, 77
Plasmodium innui
    immunity to, 118
Plasmodium knowlesi
    circadian rhythms, 22
    virulence of, 118
Plasmodium lophurae
    immunity to, 108
Plasmodium malariae
    immunity to, 118
Plasmodium vaughani
    cross immunity, 59
Plasmodium vinckei
    immunity to, 118
Plasmodium vivax
    immunity to, 118
    life cycle, 146
Plasmodium sp.
    asexual reproduction, 22
    circadian rhythms, 22
    control of, 108
    cross immunity, 58–59
    epidemiology, 132–133

Plasmodium sp.—*cont.*
    host resistance to, 63, 108, 118
    immunity to, 108, 118
    infective stages, 22
    site of, 47
    specificity, 27, 34
    vectors (see under species)
Plerocercoid larvae, 12, 84, 98, 100
Podocotyle atomon
    host selection, 36
Podocotyle sp.
    preferred site, **46**, 47
    seasonal cycle, **99**–100
Poisson model of dispersion, 67, **68**
Polya-Aeppli model of dispersion, 67
Polymorphism of trypanosomes, 96, 115–**116**,
        117
Polymorphus minutus
    dispersal of, 13
    other species, 58
Polymorphus paradoxus
    effect on host behaviour, 21
Polystoma integerrimum
    dispersion of, 65, 67
    synchronisation with host cycle, 23, 89
Pomphorhynchus laevis
    life cycle, 147
    over dispersion, 69
    population changes, **96**–97
    specificity, 30
Population
    definition of, 1–2
    growth model of, **2**–4
Positive feedback, 3
Posthodiplostomum cuticola
    specificity, 28
Post-parturient rise, 25, 125
Predation of parasites, 57, 58
Premunition, 103, 108, 115, 118, 122
Procercoid, 12, 32, 55
Proteocephalus ambloplitis
    population changes, 100–101
Proteocephalus filicollis
    life cycle, 147
    maturation cycle, 88–89, 98, 101
    population regulation, 98, **101**
    random dispersion of, **68**
Proteocephalus fluviatilis
    population cycle, 100
Proteocephalus percae
    age distribution, 63, 64

Raillietina cesticillus
    emigration of, 49, 110
    population regulation, 110–111
Random distribution, 1, 67, **68**, 69
Recognition of hosts, 15–20
Rediae, 8, 33, 80
Reptile hosts, 67
Reservoir hosts, 133–134
Resting stages, 7, 12, 15–17, 37, 38, 84

161